Sleep Routines for Baby and You

How to Help Your Child Sleep Through the Night and Finally Get the Rest You Crave (From Newborn to School Age)

Raquel Grace

© Copyright 2020 - All rights reserved.

The content contained within this book may not be reproduced, duplicated or transmitted without direct written permission from the author or the publisher.

Under no circumstances will any blame or legal responsibility be held against the publisher, or author, for any damages, reparation, or monetary loss due to the information contained within this book, either directly or indirectly.

Legal Notice:

This book is copyright protected. It is only for personal use. You cannot amend, distribute, sell, use, quote or paraphrase any part, or the content within this book, without the consent of the author or publisher.

Disclaimer Notice:

Please note the information contained within this document is for educational and entertainment purposes only. All effort has been executed to present accurate, up to date, reliable, complete information. No warranties of any kind are declared or implied. Readers acknowledge that the author is not engaging in the rendering of legal, financial, medical or professional advice. The content within this book has been derived from various sources.

Please consult a licensed professional before attempting any techniques outlined in this book.

By reading this document, the reader agrees that under no circumstances is the author responsible for any losses, direct or indirect, that are incurred as a result of the use of information contained within this document, including, but not limited to, errors, omissions, or inaccuracies.

Table of Contents

INTRODUCTION 1
- "War and Peace" 1
- Uneasy Truce 1
- The First Baby 3
- The Value of Research 5
- Proven Sleep Training Solutions at Your Fingertips 6

CHAPTER 1: PARENTING TYPES 8
- Styles of Parenting 9
  - The Authoritarian Parent 11
  - The Authoritative or Balanced Parent 12
  - The Permissive Parent 13
  - The Uninvolved, Dismissive, or Neglectful Parent 14
- Which Parenting Style Best Suits You? 15
- Understanding Your Own Child 16
  - Sleep Temperament 16
  - Observation 17
  - Communication 18
  - Social Interaction 19
  - Physiological Milestones 19
- The Role of the Parent as Teacher 20

CHAPTER 2: HOW MUCH SLEEP IS SUFFICIENT? 22
- Sleep Recommendations 22
  - Newborn to Six Weeks 25
  - Infants - Five to Twelve Months 26
  - Toddlers - Twelve to Twenty-Four Months 27
  - Preschool - Three to Four Years 28
  - School Age - Five to Twelve Years 30

CHAPTER 3: THE MERITS OF A GOOD NIGHT'S SLEEP 32
- Busy Body, Busy Brain 33
  - What your child's brain is busy with while they are asleep. ... 34
- Grow, Body, Grow 37
- Did you know your child's body grows when they are asleep? ... 37
- A Good Night's Sleep Bolsters Your Child's Immune System 38
- The Link Between Sleep Deprivation and Overeating 39
- The Stages of Sleep 40
- How Sleep Works 41

Sleep Stage One 41
Sleep Stage Two 41
Sleep Stage Three 42
Sleep Stage Four 42

CHAPTER 4: THE VALUE OF GOOD SLEEP ROUTINES **44**

"I CAN TAKE ON THE WORLD, MOM!" 44
Ways to Encourage Healthy Sleep Habits 45
The Peaceful, Contented Child 45
The Importance of Academic Success 46
Improved Creativity 48
The Link Between Sleep and Your Child's IQ 49

CHAPTER 5: THE CAUSES OF SLEEP PROBLEMS **51**

SLEEPING PROBLEMS - YOUNG CHILDREN 52
Physical Discomfort 52
Emotional Discomfort 57
SLEEP PROBLEMS IN OLDER CHILDREN 58
Night Terrors 59
Normal Childhood Fears and Anxiety 59
Excessive Competition 60
Cyber or Social Media Bullying 61
Depression and Eating Disorders 61

CHAPTER 6: SLEEP DEPRIVATION - THE NEGATIVE IMPACT **63**

SOCIAL AND EMOTIONAL BONDS 63
INAPPROPRIATE BEHAVIOR ESCALATES 64
THE IMPACT ON SELF-ESTEEM 65
SUBSTANDARD ACADEMIC ACHIEVEMENT 66
ATTENTION-DEFICIT 67
PSYCHOSOMATIC ILLNESSES 67
INADEQUATE PHYSICAL GROWTH AND SLEEPLESSNESS 68
IMMUNE SYSTEM 68
OVERALL POOR PERFORMANCE 69

CHAPTER 7: SIGNS OF SLEEP DEPRIVATION **71**

SLEEP DISORDERS 71
Slow to Wake 72
Short Attention Span and Lack of Focus 72
Hyperactivity and Disruptive Behavior 73
Lacks Motivation 73

- *Clumsy Behavior* 73
- *Frequent Illness* 74
- *Constant Yawning* 76
- *Aggressive Behavior* 77
- *Bed-Wetting* 77
- *Snoring* 77
- *Sleepwalking or Night Terrors* 78
- *Restless Leg Syndrome* 78

CHAPTER 8: THE DANGERS OF TECHNOLOGY FOR CHILDREN 79

- THE IMPACT OF INCREASED TECHNOLOGY USE ON CHILDREN 79
- RESULTS OF THE SURVEY INTO THE USE OF TECHNOLOGY 81
- IS IT ALL NEGATIVE? 83

CHAPTER 9: POSSIBLE SOLUTIONS TO SLEEP DISRUPTION 84

- PARENTAL CONTROL 84
  - *Some Ideas to Assist Your Child in Falling Asleep Quickly* 86
  - *Sleep Training for Successful Sleep Routines* 88
- AND WHEN ALL ELSE FAILS? 93
  - *Child Psychology* 93

CONCLUSION: DON'T GIVE UP! 97

- PARENTAL EXAMPLE 97
- SLEEP ROUTINES 97
- SLEEP DEPRIVATION 99
- SLEEP DEBT 100
- QUIET SPACE 101
  - *The Importance of "Pockets of Peace"* 101
- RESOURCES FOR PARENTS 102
  - *Apps for Adults* 103
  - *Apps for Children* 107
  - *Sleep Gadgets to Help Your Child Fall Asleep* 113
  - *The Final Choice* 116

REFERENCES 118

Introduction

"War and Peace"

Most parents look forward to enjoying a happy, peaceful coexistence with their children. Realistically, however, many normal, busy homes are seldom a Utopian paradise. Parents who work long hours to support their families may find themselves too exhausted at the end of the day to make the effort to instill consistent routines and to teach their children good sleep habits. In some instances, these parents resort to taking the "easy way out" when confronted with their moody, overtired child. This is certainly an enticing option! They either attempt to cajole the child into going to bed by using bribes and when this fails, which it eventually will do, these parents give up the fight and allow their child to stay up later than is good for their well-being. The end result becomes a toss-up between an uneasy peace and outright war where the peace option is seldom victorious.

Uneasy Truce

A good sleep routine is as vital for your child's health and overall well-being as are healthy food and exercise. Chronic sleep loss lays the child open to an almost endless list of problems that would not be experienced if good sleep routines were consistently followed.

First-time parents may not realize the negative impact too little sleep can have on their child's long-term successful growth and development. The negative aspects of the "knock-on effect" of sleep deprivation for a child and the devastating consequences this is likely to have for the entire family cannot be underestimated. Imagine NO SLEEP for an endless succession of nights! NO THANK YOU! Going without an occasional good night's rest is manageable for most adults. When consecutive sleepless nights become the norm, the resulting exhaustion for both parents and their children may lead to a multitude of unpleasant and unnecessary issues. Among these, stress and anxiety rate very high. Stress is ranked as one of the deadliest causes of both physical and mental illnesses. Early indications of children suffering from sleep deprivation may be exhibited by unexpected mood swings resulting in the onset of unusual behavior patterns. In severe cases where children do not enjoy the luxury of a restful night's sleep, these children may begin to suffer from psychosomatic illnesses and may even begin to self-mutilate or contemplate suicide.

Although adults who suffer from loss of regular, peaceful sleep can continue to cope with their daily lives with some degree of functionality, children need ALL the sleep they can get in order to function at their optimal level. Children between the ages of three and six years who lack consistent, good sleep routines become moody, uncooperative and are just not so pleasant to spend time with. These children often demonstrate an increased chance of sustaining physical injuries as a result of their brain's decreased ability to correctly interpret perceptual messages. They are often too tired to take notice of stairs or obstacles in their path or realize while out riding their favorite bike that the bend in the road is sharper than they imagined. The end result—unexplained and unexpected accidents that may cause the child some major physical harm.

Other health problems in children are linked directly to lack of sleep. Many of these might be avoided if children enjoyed their full quota of between eight and ten hours of sleep each night. Senior study author Christopher Owen of St Georges' University in London (as cited in Rapaport, 2017), after the results of a study completed on children with diabetes were released, said, "These findings suggest increasing sleep duration could offer a simple, cost-effective approach to reducing levels of body fat and type 2 diabetes risk early in life." Children who suffer from less sleep are therefore more likely to develop insulin resistance. These children may also display increased body mass due to a lack of exercise and incorrect eating habits. According to the American Academy of Pediatrics (2014), insufficient sleep is closely linked to high blood pressure, obesity, depression and an increase in the likelihood of accidents. It is therefore essential for parents to institute good sleep routines as early as possible in their child's life. The development of good sleeping habits can assist children in falling asleep MORE quickly and being able to enjoy sleeping for longer periods.

The First Baby

WE ARE EXPECTING! What a happy announcement, full of excitement and expectation. The arrival of the first baby can be exciting, and in some cases, quite a daunting experience for parents. New parents do not know what to expect, and so many of them read copious amounts of literature on the subjects of birthing and rearing their new "bundle of joy." With so much information available, where does the new parent begin? Apart from the feeding and diaper changing routines, there is the all-important quality parent-child interaction time. This tiny, new person who initially dictates their every need, relies solely on their parents for the satisfaction of their physical requirements. Later, as they grow and matures they demand guidance and instruction in order to reach their full potential on their journey to becoming a successful and fully integrated member of society.

Perhaps one of the very first milestones they will need to conquer is the establishment of a good sleep routine. Sound, restful sleep forms the foundation for a happy, healthy, and successful life.

As with the acquisition of all new skills, most are either taught while others are learned through mimicking an example. The importance of the parental role cannot be overemphasized. Through maintaining consistent, although not necessarily rigid, routines at home, parents can assist their baby to feel sufficiently secure and comfortable to sleep at regular intervals during the day. This sleep pattern will include naps where necessary as well as the normal nighttime sleep. If good, healthy sleep habits are instilled early enough in the child, these are likely to continue for his entire lifetime.

The author of *Healthy Sleep Habits, Happy Child, 4th Edition: A Step-By-Step Program for a Good Night's Sleep,* Dr. Marc Weissbluth (2015), explains your child's sleep patterns are a reliable indicator of their overall quality of life. The baby's first year is the most important because it is during these twelve months that the child establishes a good sleep routine as early sleep training sets the pattern for long-term successful sleep. It is important for parents to remember that their baby should not reach a stage of being overtired before they are encouraged to sleep. Young children do not fall asleep easily when they become overtired. The reverse is in fact true. When a good sleep routine is established, the baby is put into their cot at approximately the same time each night. The better the routine, the sooner the baby falls asleep and the longer the period of rest the child enjoys. However, Dr. Weissbluth does not advocate a rigid routine. He believes that because no two babies are exactly alike, it is essential to take the child's temperament into account when training sleep routines.

According to Nicole Johnson, founder and lead sleep consultant of The Baby Sleep Site, (Johnson, 2019a), the assumption that Dr. Weissbluth makes about all babies needing to sleep for at least twelve hours straight is unrealistic. She suggests each baby is an individual who will develop their own sleeping routine according to their own needs. and believes very early bedtimes for babies are not always practical for modern working parents. Flexibility is the key.

The Value of Research

According to a number of well-researched studies conducted by the Douglas Research Centre (n.d.), there is a definable link between the contribution a good, restful night's sleep makes to most aspects of our physical, mental and emotional well-being. Consistent lack of sleep has a similar effect on our bodies and brains as overindulging in alcohol. Researchers of sleep deprivation and related problems suggest that "poor sleep may directly affect" increased sensitivity to pain and may well negatively affect the development of "cardiovascular problems."

Children who enjoy their sufficient quota of sleep are more content. They generally develop improved attention and memory skills and cope better with academic tasks at school. These children are also more likely to demonstrate enhanced learning ability as well as emotional and social skills. Children with good sleep routines are usually more independent and enthusiastic to explore their environment. They may also learn to walk and talk sooner, which gives them a substantial advantage over their sleep-deprived counterparts.

Proven Sleep Training Solutions at Your Fingertips

You may well wonder why the need for another book on the topic of healthy sleeping habits? *The Happy Healthy Sleeper – Proven Sleep Training Solutions to Help Your Baby Sleep Deeply Through the Night and Save Time and Tears (From Newborn to School Age)* is a useful resource book filled with valuable information and advice for parents who wish to establish good, consistent sleep routines. The easy-to-read format and comfortable, homely style of the writing is sure to encourage parents to feel right at home as they begin their journey towards discovering proven sleep training solutions for their overactive, sleepless children.

This book offers parents who struggle with a child who neither falls asleep easily nor remains peacefully asleep for any reasonable length of time, beneficial advice they can apply to establish healthy, sleep routines to overcome the challenges of their sleep-deprived child.

Most families who live in the rush and bustle of the 21st century suffer to some degree from sleep deprivation. The fact that we are more electronically active than our own parents play an important role in our current everyday lifestyle. Children are often more comfortable and enthusiastic about operating electronic devices than playing outdoors. Added to this sedentary way of life is the lack of good, dependable home routines.

The Happy Healthy Sleeper – Proven Sleep Training Solutions to Help Your Baby Sleep Deeply Through the Night and Save Time and Tears (From Newborn to School Age) offers supportive ideas to overcome the challenge of the sleep-deprived child and assist parents in formulating a good sleep routine, without fuss and drama. A great deal of research has already been done on the importance of developing and maintaining good sleeping habits for young children. There is a definite link between children with poor-quality sleep patterns and underachievement at school. Badly behaved children with low self-esteem and an aggressive attitude may well be the victims of sleep deprivation, which has largely gone unnoticed.

Chapter 1: Parenting Types

A parent's duty to their children is of paramount importance and should be taken seriously. Prior to the baby's arrival, parents will have made a conscious, committed decision to shoulder their responsibilities to their "little bundle of joy" and to undertake to raise them to the very best of their abilities.

Besides setting good examples, this fundamental obligation to the child also involves an understanding of the importance of the implementation of consistent rules, boundaries, and routines in the home. Parents are their child's initial, and perhaps most important, teacher. This role comes with an enormous amount of responsibility and should never be taken lightly. The child looks to their parents for guidance, reassurance, and the knowledge of what behavior is appropriate and acceptable and notification of what is not. Some psychologists believe children feel more secure when they have a clear understanding of what is expected of them. Parents who set fair and reasonable parameters for their children assist them to learn and work cooperatively within these boundaries. All children need boundaries in order to function at their optimum level.

An enormous amount of debate arises out of the issue of discipline. The most up-to-date research shows the positive impact rules, boundaries, and routines have for optimum development of the child's full potential.

Styles of Parenting

Although much has been written and spoken about the good and bad aspects of raising children, there is, in fact, no single parenting handbook that can address every potential pitfall in this sometimes overwhelming business of parenting.

A number of parenting styles have been promulgated, each of which has value as well as some flaws. Depending on the parent's personal preference, either one specific style may be chosen, or an accumulation of ideas from a variety of styles may be considered. As with every child having been gifted with an individual personality, each parent has their own personal style of parenting. This style may mirror their own childhood experiences, both good and bad, or it may be a conglomeration of the advice from family members and friends. Some parents take their role more seriously than others and will research as much information as possible on raising and educating their child as successfully as possible. Other parents demonstrate a more formal approach to child-rearing while a third group prefers a more "laid-back" attitude to the business of parenting.

There is no right or wrong style of parenting. A good general rule is to carefully consider the style that works best for each individual parent and their child. This may result in the parents choosing suitable aspects from a number of different styles in order to create their own unique method of tackling this sometimes controversial issue of effectively raising children.

The best advice any parent can receive is firstly, always do their best for their child. Parents are encouraged to put their child's best interests first and take responsibility for their role as parents. Also, remember that your child is an individual in their own right and needs to be treated as such.

Secondly, parents should try to remain consistent in their decisions and expedite rules and routines that have a positive outcome for their child.

Thirdly, and perhaps most importantly, parents need to DUMP THE GUILT they may be carrying. The more parents read and learn, the guiltier they sometimes begin to feel because they allow external influences to cloud their judgments and force them into believing they are inadequate parents and role models for the children. The confusion this can sometimes cause can make parents worry unduly about whether or not they have this "parenting business" under control.

Parents generally know a great deal about their own children and family structure from the inside, so to speak. Visitors, those family members who do not live under the same roof, and members of the community may only have knowledge of the exterior view of the family. These "outsiders" are not always fairly or justifiably equipped to comment on how best parents should raise their children.

This being said, there are however some basic, common responsibilities that apply to all families irrespective of their economic or social status. Parents are legally bound to care for their children to the best of their abilities and to provide their families with a safe living environment. They are expected to love and nurture their children, providing shelter, food, and clothing. Over and above those mentioned, another vitally important responsibility that is often overlooked is the important duty of parents to create sensible boundaries for behavior and to develop good, consistent routines for their children.

Diana Baumrind (Positive-Parenting-Ally, n.d.), a well-known psychologist in the 1960's, studied 100 children of preschool age and discovered a number of interesting facts about parenting styles. From her results, she identified three distinct ways in which parents raise their children. A fourth, more progressive style was added to the list by Maccoby and Martin.

Diana Baumrind used two diagnostic evaluation devices to assess parenting styles. The first of these, Parental Responsiveness vs. Parental Unresponsiveness, measures the level of parental interaction and response. Her second evaluation device measured Parental Demandingness vs. Parental Undemandingness, which in a nutshell refers to the parents' ability and willingness to exercise control over their children's behavior.

The parenting styles discussed here, may be described as "models" as they offer rigid examples of parenting styles and the expected responses. Most parents make use of a combination of styles in order to cope with the individual personalities of each of their children.

The Authoritarian Parent

This strict parenting style is often considered very old-fashioned and has been proven to have a long-term, detrimental effect on some of the children raised this way. Parents who make use of this authoritarian approach are dictatorial and imperious. Their austere parenting approach generally creates a great deal of unnecessary stress and resentment in their children. Household and family rules are strictly enforced by these parents without any deviation permitted, and any transgressions are usually met with more stringent rules and in some cases, harsh punishments. Authoritarian parents have high expectations for their children but seldom show warmth, nurturing, or understanding. They seldom support their children with advice and direction, expecting them to behave in an exemplary manner as 'mini-adults.'

Children raised with this style of parenting may become cowardly and fearful. They have low self-esteem and seldom show the desire to tackle new challenges or use their own initiative for fear of making errors. These children may appear outwardly obedient and display 'model behavior' as their low response to the high demands of their parents. However, the resentment they may harbor towards their overbearing parents may fester over time and develop into behavioral disorders in later life.

The Authoritative or Balanced Parent

This type of parenting style is perhaps the most positive and productive. Parents using this balanced approach to raising their children show them copious amounts of love, support, and understanding. They generally take a keen interest in every aspect of their child's life and encourage their children to exercise their own judgment and make their own choices based on the sensible options provided.

These parents make use of open, transparent, and clearly

conveyed communication to discuss solutions to potential or perceived problems. They promote and endorse two-way communication as a cooperative way of sharing ideas.

Honesty, integrity, and respectful behavior are encouraged by the parents setting good examples for their children to mimic. Although these parents offer their children support to develop independently according to their individual abilities, they are always on hand to offer advice and support when required. These parents are usually considered to demonstrate a "hands-on" parenting style, and they are well aware of their responsibilities for raising successful, well-balanced children. They seldom sidestep their duty to their children and are proud to retain their parental role no matter what, under any and every circumstance.

Children raised by authoritative parents are generally well-balanced and happy. They are confident and enjoy accepting challenges. Instead of being punished, they learn through their mistakes. These children exhibit a high response to the high demand of their parents and they usually cope well academically and socially because they are self-confident and capable individuals.

The Permissive Parent

This parenting style is characterized by high responses and low demands. Although these parents are often loving and very caring, they have few expectations for their children. They generally prefer to neither set boundaries nor instill routines, and they tend to encourage their children to do as they please.

These permissive parents may be referred to as being

overindulgent of their children. They seldom make use of many forms of discipline, and their children have no guidelines or boundaries. Parents who enjoy this style of parenting communicate well with their children, often showering them with affection but emphasizing their preference of being their child's friend rather than the parent.

Children raised by permissive parents often experience difficulty settling into school routines and accepting authority. They are more likely to throw tantrums and often backtalk their parents and other adults. These children have a poor understanding of social etiquette, and they are often unpopular with their peers. They are difficult to control because of their disregard for authority coupled with their unwillingness to work cooperatively within expected boundaries. These children display a high response to their parent's low demand and are often considered socially impaired because they generally do as they please without any regard for the consequences of their actions.

The Uninvolved, Dismissive, or Neglectful Parent

This type of "hands-off" parenting style devalues the child's sense of worth because the parent takes the approach that the child comes second to all of the other activities in which the parent is involved. Although uninvolved parents may take good care of their child's physical needs, they serious neglect their emotional prerequisites. They offer no support or guidance to their children. They seldom interact with their children and are dismissive of their children's efforts. Communication is usually kept to a minimum, and family conversation is restricted to providing basic information.

Children raised by neglectful parents quickly learn that their own challenges and achievements are of little interest to their parents. Beyond essential information, they seldom share ideas or information with their parents and tend to become independent fairly soon in life. These children exhibit a low response to the low demands made by their parents and may either develop a fixation on overachieving both academically and socially in order to prove their own self-worth, or they lose interest altogether in striving for success and develop nothing more than mediocre skills.

Which Parenting Style Best Suits You?

So, which of these parenting styles will best suit you? To make the right decision, you need to bear in mind that parenting styles are as unique as the parents themselves, and no two children respond identically to the same style of parenting. Individual parenting styles result in a noticeably specific behavior pattern in their children.

The authoritative parenting style is perhaps the most socially acceptable because of its more caring and balanced approach to raising children. Children whose parents advocate this style are taught the importance of rules and routines and are given the opportunity to interact with their parents in order to internalize what they have learned. Authoritative parents treat their children fairly and with respect. In return, their children are courteous and cooperative, not out of fear, but out of an understanding of the value of rules, routines, and boundaries within which they live happily.

Understanding Your Own Child

Understanding your own children's individual personalities and their needs is of paramount importance to every parent's successful implementation of their parenting skills. In other words, perhaps the most important advice a parent can receive is to learn to understand their own child as an individual and seriously consider what will work best for them in the long run. Every parent aspires to raise happy, well-adjusted children who will be academically and socially successful. It is only when parents take the time to really get to know their child's personal characteristics and idiosyncrasies that they will find their parenting role truly fulfilling.

Sleep Temperament

Each child is born with their own individual personality, despite their socio-economic situation. These personal characteristics are noticeable in the way the baby eats, drinks, and how they respond to their parents with a smile or a frown. They also begin to develop a 'sleep pattern' which can be termed the child's sleep temperament.

Two specific and very different types of sleep temperament have been identified, namely sleep-soothers and signalers.

Self-Soothers

These little children have the ability to settle themselves and drop back to sleep without much fuss. They generally doze off for regular naps throughout the day and are often classed as "easy babies." Self-soothers are not as dependent on their parents for sleep support as signalers.

Signalers

Babies that fit into this category are the ones who need, and in fact, demand attention from their parents during the night. They are often difficult to settle at bedtime as they require more creative ways to encourage them to relax and go off to sleep. They are also unable to return to sleep without some added support and encouragement. These babies may respond to rocking or cuddling, and when they see their parents enter the room in response to their yelling, their little faces often light up with a beatific smile. Hard for most parents to resist, even when they are dragging their own feet from sheer exhaustion! The challenge with the signalers is that parents can so easily fall prey to the child's demands, and in next to no time, sleep time becomes a nightmare of demand and respond.

Although there is no cut-and-dried rule for what will work for your baby, consistent, routine sleep-time patterns should be encouraged as early as possible. However, successful sleeping routines really depend on a variety of factors, all of which require fair consideration.

Observation

The best way for a parent to get to know their children is through careful, daily observation. Although there are several suggested steps to follow in order to ensure this process is a success, there is no hard-and-fast rule and parents should exercise their individual common sense.

Parents should take the time to observe their children in as many aspects of their life as possible. Notice the food, games, animals, books, music, and songs they enjoy. They should find out if they are afraid of the dark, or if they are a brave "warrior" child who takes chances. Parents should take note of every detail about their child and use this information to formulate good parenting strategies and improve their parenting skills.

Whatever sleep temperament your child displays, it is important to observe the pattern and then decide on a suitable course of action. Do not assume the sleep temperament is permanent. Oh, no! As your baby grows and develops, their sleep temperament may change. When this happens, which it probably will, parents should accept the change and "go with the flow."

Communication

Parents are reminded that good communication is the key to any successful relationship. The bond between parent and child is perhaps the most important of its kind that a parent will ever construct. Younger children usually respond positively to a calm approach and gentle words of support. Older children should be encouraged to talk about their fears, worries, and hopes so that parents can offer support and advice. Parents who talk to their children and give them the opportunity to answer lay the foundation for the development of good communication skills for later in their child's life.

Social Interaction

Parents should observe their children interacting with family members and friends. Listen to the child's conversations without eavesdropping, and notice their body language and mannerisms when interacting with other people. Observe if the child acts independently in a group, or perhaps they prefer to take a back seat rather than participate. Does the child prefer to lead or follow?

Physiological Milestones

Parents should be aware of the physiological milestones their child should be reaching and take their level of maturity into account. This will guide your understanding of their capabilities and allow you to set reasonable and fair expectations for your child.

No matter which style of parenting works best for you, always remember your child is a precious individual with the right to be taught the correct information that will empower and assist them to grow and develop to their optimum potential in order to become an active, integrated, and valued member of the community.

The importance of the role parents play in their children's lives cannot and should never be underestimated. Besides the legal responsibilities every parent has to their child, parents are also the primary role models their children will first use to help them learn many of the important skills needed to function correctly in real-life social and emotional situations. All children initially mimic the example set by their parents. They learn positive and negative behavior patterns in this way. Parents should be willing to step up and take responsibility for this important role they play in their child's life and realize parenting embraces continuous, active participation in your child's life.

The Role of the Parent as Teacher

Parents, as the child's primary caregivers from birth, also fulfill the role of the child's first teacher. It, therefore, behooves parents to not only be the best role models for their children but to also lay the rules and set up good routines to provide the best foundation for successful learning opportunities.

For a new baby, the world is a huge, unknown, overwhelming and unexplored place waiting to be discovered. By setting sensible, age-appropriate boundaries for their little one, parents encourage the child to explore and learn in a safe and manageable space.

As the baby becomes a toddler, a number of previously successful boundaries are likely to fall away and be replaced by new routines and limits. Each new stage of the child's development requires parents to restructure some of the "ground rules." Why is this necessary? It is important to realize that as the child develops, matures, and shows an increasing interest and desire for acquiring knowledge and improving their skills, they require increased input and explanation about their environment and how best to interact with it. The child will usually turn to their parents for information and advice.

So, why the need for this talk about rules and routines? Well quite simply, in order for people to interact socially and live cooperatively, it is important to have rules and routines that lay the foundation for these behaviors. Our lives are therefore governed by rules in one form or another. Without these rules, chaos will reign!

It is recommended that children find comfort in rules and routines. When they know and understand their boundaries, they show greater confidence to experiment, explore, and learn within the structured environment their parents have created. This is not to say that rules hamper development. On the contrary, it is believed consistent routines not only bring comfort and security to the child, but they also encourage exploration and help to develop creativity. It is believed that children who have a good foundation with consistent routines and boundaries generally develop faster. Among the usual routines for getting up in the morning, mealtimes, playtimes, homework, and leisure time, is the all-important sleep routine.

Most parents will admit to having some routines in place. They generally agree the necessity for having rules and boundaries is to maintain peace and harmony in a smooth-running home. These family rules and routines should have as one of their end goals, the happy, peaceful, and successful cooperative living of all members in the household.

Chapter 2: How Much Sleep Is Sufficient?

"Mom, I'm too tired to finish my homework!" Is this a familiar-sounding refrain in your household? Indeed, many parents can attest to the constant struggle they have to encourage their "tired" child to complete a task. Why are so many children suffering from the "I'm too tired" syndrome?

According to research completed at the Douglas Research Centre (n.d.), it has been shown that it is essential to "set aside enough time to get an adequate amount of sleep." There is no set rule for the amount of sleep your child requires to perform optimally and to remain healthy and active. Sleep is an individual process, and some children require noticeably more rest than others. However, a good rule of thumb is to plan bedtime before the child becomes overtired.

Many children find sleep comes naturally and quickly when there is a good routine in place, and parents act in a consistent manner at bedtime. Other children may struggle to switch off their thoughts and their memories of all the activities in which they participated during the day. Children who are overtired generally have difficulty falling asleep easily. The brain's ability to begin to "shut down" at sleep time is simply the body's way of giving notice of its intention to go into a state of rest. This sleep pattern strategy is vital for a good night's restful sleep.

Sleep Recommendations

Welcoming a new baby into your home is both an exciting as

well as a daunting experience. The first item on the new agenda, is more often than not, a dynamic shift in the parents' sleep patterns. No matter how challenging this diverse change in the restful nights' parents have enjoyed thus far, the new arrival will initially impose his own sleeping routine on his parents. Added to this are the demands of our hectic, modern life that directly influence families' lifestyles and sleeping routines and patterns. Many well-meaning parents living this hectic lifestyle and are caught up in their daily grind, which forces both parents out into the working world. This often results in their children being raised in crèches or day-care centers. A working parent's day usually starts early and ends late. Parents may not get to spend as much time with their children as they might wish. In scenarios such as this, routines are of vital importance; one major drawback, however, is the feeling of guilt that working parents may experience.

Children of different ages in the same family can also pose sleep routine challenges. There are a number of different beliefs about the importance of sleep routines, and what may work for one family may be disastrous for another. The development of routine sleep patterns should be established earlier in the child's life rather than later. As many studies show, the best support and preparation for life apart from a happy, secure home life that a parent can provide is to establish for your child a consistent sleep routine and all other successes should follow. Good routines that are in place from the child's early years lay the foundation for continued sleeping success.

Children of different ages do not require the same number of hours of sleep. The following amounts of sleep are suggested for optimal health and physical growth of children between birth and eighteen years of age. This includes naps as well as nighttime sleep. The table below should be viewed only as a guideline and should not be expected to be rigidly enforced.

- Infants birth to 12 months: 12 to 16 hours
- Children 1 to 2 years: 11 to 14 hours
- Children 3 to 5 years: 10 to 13 hours
- Children 6 to 12 years: 9 to 12 hours
- Teenagers 13 to 18 years: 8 to 10 hours

This author wholeheartedly concurs that when regular, adequate sleep is enjoyed by children in each of the above age groups, these children demonstrate a noticeable improvement in their mental, emotional, and physical health. Early sleep training, although it can take some time to establish, is beneficial to both parents and their children and allows the entire family to enjoy a better quality of life.

As previously mentioned, reports children who experience regular, depleted sleep patterns struggle with a number of problems associated with the sleep-deprived syndrome, including but not limited to, an increase in injuries, depression, hypertension, and in severe cases self-mutilation and suicide.

The most important data acquired from the above research undeniably proves that sleep recommendations for children differ according to their age, stage of development, as well as their own personal needs. It is, however, important to realize these suggestions act only as a guideline to assist parents with the establishment of a good sleep routine for their own individual child. As every household differs in size and nature, so too do its occupants. There is no "one-size-fits-all" solution to the conundrum of sleep routines. However, the onus rests with the parents to do the best they can to create a comfortable, workable solution for their own particular child.

Newborn to Six Weeks

To begin with, these small people set their own sleep routine which parents are encouraged to initially follow. Newborn babies can sleep up to 14 hours a day and only wake for feeding and for a diaper change.

During these first few weeks of the baby's life, there is no need for the parent to try to establish a sleep routine as the baby will dictate when they are hungry or uncomfortable. Crying is their only way of alerting their parents to their needs. With their speedy response to the baby's signal for food or comfort, parents often find they drift back to sleep quite quickly. It's important to remember not to force your baby awake for a feed. Some schools of thought believe babies should be fed every two to three hours. Unless your little one is seriously not gaining sufficient mass, it is best to let them dictate their own feeding schedule during these first few weeks of their life. As your baby grows and matures, their sleep-wake routine begins to change as do their feeding schedule and demands for attention.

Infants - Five to Twelve Months

There is a noticeable change in children around the age of three months when they begin to take a keen interest in their surroundings. They become more alert to sounds and sights and begin to recognize familiar faces and voices to which they generally respond with enthusiasm.

By the time the child is around five months of age, parents should be feeling sufficiently confident to make a concerted effort to start training their child into a good sleep routine. Children of this age are becoming more mobile as their physical strength increases. They begin to roll, kick with enthusiasm, grasp items within their reach, and generally take an even greater interest in their surrounds. These activities stimulate the brain, which in turn begins to process and store all the new information for future retrieval when required. Between five and twelve months of age, the child becomes aware of the difference between day and night and should be ready to begin a good sleep routine. Due to their regularity, routines play an important role in encouraging your child to develop a sense of security, and they begin to understand the concept of what happens next. For many children, this familiarity has a reassuring and calming effect as they become aware that their parents are in control and all is well.

Due to the increased energy required during this period of your child's growth and development program, they will require at least two daily naps and a minimum of 12 hours of sleep per 24-hour cycle. The optimum time for bed should be around 7 p.m. However, this is not a rigid rule, but rather a guideline as each family will need to adjust the time to suit their own personal way of life. Consistent, loving reinforcement of your child's sleep routine is of paramount importance to its success and should be instituted as early as possible, in order to ensure long-term sleeping success.

It is a good idea to begin the sleep routine training by encouraging the child to sleep in their own bed. The familiarity of their surroundings adds to their comfort and feelings of safety and security. Parents should be mindful now of the importance of being consistent in their efforts to develop the sleep routine. This can at times be quite challenging to stick to, but hang in there and good results will begin to show!

The key to accessing the child's hidden ability is through the parent. Whether the child realizes their full capabilities will depend on the importance their parent places on encouraging and supporting them in their endeavors. One of the most important ways a parent can help the child is to develop good routines in the home, one of which should be a consistent sleep routine.

Toddlers - Twelve to Twenty-Four Months

Oh, boy! These youngsters are always on the go, day in and day out. They are ultra-active and enthusiastic about exploring their world and learning new skills. These busybodies are absorbing crazy amounts of stimuli received through their senses of taste, touch, smell, sight, and hearing. This process happens every second of every day! Imagine, just for a second, being in their tiny shoes! The average parent wouldn't last more than an hour, absorbing and processing the same volume of information before they collapsed in an exhausted heap! Now imagine the sheer overload of information bombarding your child's brain. No wonder they get tired and sometimes cranky! Add to the mix, the fact that your toddler is more than likely in the thick of teething, which in itself, is no joke!

Okay! So, just when you thought you had the sleep routine down pat, "Whoopity-Doo!" your toddler has great news for you! Initially, parents may be nonplussed by their child's about-face and may lose hope of ever establishing a good sleep routine. It's back to the drawing board and time to rethink your strategy as you plan a new course of action. Who said parenting was a walk in the park?

This age group usually enjoys at least one nap during the day, but by 7 p.m. they should be ready for a good, sound sleep of between 12 to 14 hours. Now is the time for parents to reestablish the initial sleep routine and remain steadfastly consistent in their endeavors and reinforce this. Try different tactics while remaining focused on your goal of keeping your child calm and getting them ready for bed as soon as possible.

A warm bath and perhaps a massage may help. Reading a short bedtime story or encouraging your child to talk about the pictures in their favorite book may ease them into a more relaxed frame of mind. Soft music and dim lighting may add to the calm ambiance of the room and before you know it, your toddler is fast asleep.

Preschool - Three to Four Years

Preschool children offer their parents a different set of challenges. These children are busier than their younger counterparts, more vocal, and can sometimes become quite bossy. Between the age of three and four years, children are developing a keen awareness of their own independence and many begin to consciously wield power over their siblings and parents. You may hear the refrain, "Leave me! I can do this!" from this age group. Their cute antics sometimes cause parents to lose sight of the bigger picture and yield to their demands, especially at bedtime. Now is the time to stand steadfast in your resolve as a parent and stick to the sleep routine as if your life depended on it, which in some respects it sure does!

Sleep routines that appeared to be well-entrenched once again undergo the need for some adjustment and tweaking. Now maybe the time for the parent to indulge in a delightful bedtime story or perhaps prayer time, before the final cuddle and good night kiss.

It is important to bear in mind that children of this age and stage of development live in a fantasy world. They may begin to suffer from night terrors and anxiety, which has its roots in specific incidents that occurred during the day. They may require a great deal of reassurance before they drop off to sleep. Parents should be aware consistent reinforcement of good sleep routines should continue despite this emotional war being waged between parent and child.

Avoid scary movies and stories. Encourage your child to chat about the day's events. Ask leading questions in order to elicit information. Say something like, "What did you build in the sandpit at school?" or "Who was your favorite friend at school today?" Help them to verbalize incidents that upset them as well as those that made them feel happy.

Preschool children generally love bedtime stories, and some may even want to "read" their own story aloud. Encourage this interest as it will forever foster a love of reading for life.

Parents can build in some very valuable personal relaxation time during their child's sleep routine. Often, just the fact of being together with your child in this one-on-one state is enough to unwind after a hectic day at the office. No matter how tempting, don't fall asleep on the job though!

School Age - Five to Twelve Years

If these school-going children have not enjoyed good sleep routines from a young age, they generally struggle to fall asleep and often end up suffering from a severe lack of rest. Strict bedtime routines for this age group are difficult to enforce due to often extensive homework schedules and sporting commitments. The secret is to ensure there is some sort of routine in place and that there is still room for non-negotiable rules. One of these should perhaps include the removal of all electronic devices from the bedroom. These will include, the television, laptop, smartphone, and tablet. Extended use of these devices is proven to have a detrimental effect on the child's brain and upsets the body's internal clock by suppressing the release of a valuable hormone called melatonin. This hormone regulates the child's sleeping pattern. The blue light emitted by these electronic devices interferes with normal brain waves by stimulating it into a wakeful state which delays the onset of the essential stage of REM sleep. With continued use of these devices before bedtime, the long-term effects of sleep deprivation caused will have a lasting detrimental outcome for the child's emotional and social well-being, not to mention the negative impact on their scholastic success.

A second good option to consider for these children is to encourage them to read before going to sleep. This "old-fashioned" practice helps the child develop improved language skills by training visual discrimination and visual accuracy, both of which have a positive impact on improving comprehension skills.

Primary school children require between 9 and 10 hours of sleep every night because they often participate in exceptionally busy school and sport routines that keep them on the go during waking hours. These children expend vast amounts of energy learning new physical and intellectual skills, tackling cognitive challenges, expanding their vocabulary, and developing socially.

Children of school-going age, who already have well-established good sleep routines, automatically continue to enjoy a restful night's sleep. Studies show primary school children can improve their academic performance by increasing their daily sleep routine time by as little as 30 minutes. Good, well-entrenched sleep routines are vitally important for these children to ensure they continue to enjoy healthy, happy lives and have every possible opportunity to reach their full potential in all aspects.

Chapter 3: The Merits of a Good Night's Sleep

Kimberley Hardin, MD, director of the sleep fellowship program at the University of California, Davis, (as cited in Hochron, 2016) reports that "people underestimate the importance of sleep." Sleep deprivation is on the increase in modern society and is directly linked to lifestyle choices.

It is important to remember that every living creature requires routine periods of rest in order to successfully grow and survive. Your baby is no exception.

In the early stages of their life, your child learns quickly to summon their parents when they experience hunger, thirst, or physical discomfit. As they grow and they begin to mature, they respond to the natural indicators given off in their brain that encourage them to roll and move forward, make sounds, and grasp items.

All these activities require energy and are quite literally exhausting for your tiny baby. During waking hours, the body produces increased amounts of a hormone known as adrenaline. This hormone keeps the body in a state of readiness for "fight or flight" situations. The longer the child stays awake, the more adrenaline is secreted, the more active the child and the less likely they are to sleep well.

As previously stated, in many instances, your child will take a number of naps during the day. These periods of rest, no matter how short they may be, give them the opportunity to recharge their brain and body for the next round of exploration and learning. For the majority of very young children between the ages of birth and three months, these periods of sleep may be quite regular, to begin with and sufficiently long to allow for the body and mind the chance to enjoy a good rest. There are, however, always exceptions to the rule. These are the children who bewilder their parents because they are difficult to train into any good routines, let alone sleep through the night. So, the challenge with these little ones is patience and consistent reinforcement of sleep routines. As noted in Chapter 8: Possible Solutions to Sleep Disruptions, a number of positive suggestions are available for the children who find it difficult to wind down and fall asleep easily.

Suzanne Stevens, MD, a sleep neurologist at the University of Kansas Health System, (The University of Kansas Health System, n.d.), believes "chronic poor sleep affects the ability to function well." Without good quality rest, our bodies cannot function properly, resulting in a variety of unpleasant side effects. Many of these are discussed in Chapter 6: The Negative Impact of Sleep Deprivation on Children. In order to function at their optimal best and grow to their full potential, it is therefore essential for your child to enjoy sufficient, good quality sleep.

Busy Body, Busy Brain

The brain is one of the first organs to develop in the fetus. It begins to grow and develop in earnest before birth and continues well into early childhood. When your child enjoys consistent quality sleep, their mental, emotional, and physical performance automatically improves. Good sleep is proven to have a positive impact on their immune system while simultaneously balancing hormones, boosting metabolism, and improving their overall brain function.

What your child's brain is busy with while they are asleep.

According to Dr. Stevens (The University of Kansas Health System, n.d.), as referenced above, the main reason sleep is so important for your child's success in school is because, during the sleep process, his brain has an opportunity to "clean" itself and toss out all the "brain garbage," Brain cells, like every other cell in your child's body, are living, consuming food, and reproducing. While your child is awake, his brain is in "super active" mode, busy with exploring and learning, thinking, and figuring out new information, explains Dr. Stevens. The brain controls your child's body and all the functions it completes daily. All this activity creates a heap of "brain garbage," which in fact is no longer viable or useful and takes up valuable space and is in fact needed for the storage of new information.

During sleep, your child's body makes good use of this period of rest to remove all the waste that has built up during the day and then it starts the entire process of storing new information, from scratch. This activity can be compared to when you dump all your unwanted computer files into the recycle bin, ready for disposal in order to make room for more new information. According to Jake Gamsky (2016), if your child is not getting sufficient quality sleep, this "brain garbage" begins to back up in the brain and starts clogging the system and reducing your child's cognitive performance and learning potential.

The complex process known as sleep plays a vital role in our lives. The director of the Systems Neurobiology Laboratory at the University of Toronto, John Peever, and the director of the sleep laboratory at the Sunnybrook Health Sciences Center, Brian J. Murray, (Scientific American, 2015), believe that during your child's sleep cycle, this essential brain refueling process, which is, in fact, the backbone for the control of all learning and the development of optimum memory, is activated. Sleep is also known to play an important role in appetite control (see the information in Chapter 5: The Causes of Sleep Problems) as well as being a major factor for balancing your child's emotions and keeping them cheerful.

Scientists have discovered the brain generates two different types of sleep. The first type of sleep is what is known as Slow Wave Sleep (SWS). Slow Wave Sleep generates deep, slow breathing and a definite decrease in your child's heart rate and pulse. It is during these periods of Slow Wave Sleep that the brain recuperates, recharges, and readies itself in preparation for the challenges of a new day.

The second type of sleep is known as Rapid Eye Movement (REM) sleep, during which stage it is believed your child experiences dreams. Both these types of sleep are discussed in more detail later in this chapter.

During wakefulness, the body is in a constantly active state. Vast amounts of stimuli are received from the child's immediate environment. These stimuli are collected via the child's senses of sight and hearing, taste, touch, and smell. The brain, which is in control of all bodily functions, as well as all movements, thought processes, and emotions remain constantly alert to process these millions of physical, emotional, perceptual, and academic messages the body receives every second.

As the child grows and learns new skills, his "information bank" begins to increase. These memory processes utilize a great deal of energy. This can be an exhausting process, as any parent who has experienced learning a new skill themselves will attest to it. The process of storing all this new information, known in scientific terms as "assimilation," occurs during the time your baby is asleep and his little body is enjoying this period of rest, the brain can concentrate as it were, on "brain matters" only, instead of being required to focus on all the other activities that wakeful children enjoy. Interrupted sleep is proven to have a negative impact on this process of assimilation of information. Consistent disruption during this sorting and storing process is likely to be responsible for the loss of information and the incorrect processing or adequate storing of important data. This unfinished business can become the forerunner for future learning and concentration challenges for your little one.

The value of good sleep routines cannot be overemphasized! With a well-rested body and brain, your child is ready to take on and conquer the world. If sleep then is one of the basic building blocks for good health, it stands to reason that parents should try at all costs to ensure their children enjoy regular restful sleep by establishing a good sleeping routine as early as possible.

Grow, Body, Grow

Did you know your child's body grows when they are asleep?

There is empirical evidence that a child's body undergoes multiple growth spurts while it is in a period of undisturbed, deep rest. A vital hormone found in the pituitary gland, known as Human Growth Hormone (HGH), is released into the child's bloodstream during sleep stage three, which is when the body is in a deep, restful sleep.

This growth hormone is essential for your child's optimum growth and good physical health. The primary value of the Human Growth Hormone lies in its ability to restore damaged cells and repair injured body tissue. The release of this important growth hormone begins when your baby is very young, and it peaks around the time they reach puberty. As we age, the Human Growth Hormone begins to decrease.

The importance of the value of the Human Growth Hormone to your child cannot be underestimated, as it is one of the major building blocks in your child's body responsible for encouraging the development of a healthy metabolism while simultaneously enhancing your child's physical performance.

A Good Night's Sleep Bolsters Your Child's Immune System

The task of the human immune system is to protect your child's body against the harmful and damaging infiltration and influence of viruses that cause many different illnesses. This can be compared to having their own private internal security system guarding them against potential dangers and unexpected onslaughts. A number of different studies have been done on the value of good, regular, restful sleep has for the child's immune system. Stoyan Dimitrov, PhD, a German researcher at the University of Tubingen (Rockefeller University Press, 2019), discovered that consistently good sleep routines positively affect the growth of very important pathogen-fighting (disease-fighting) cells known as T-cells.

While we are awake and active, stress hormones such as adrenaline suppress these T-cells and interfere with their ability to fight disease. However, during periods of deep, restful sleep, these T-cells "power up" their sticky coat as soon as they receive an indication from the brain of the presence of disease-causing cells in the body, such as cancer and viruses. These T-cells rush out and adhere to the enemy cells and annihilate them. That sounds like the best way to dispose of these unwanted enemies!

Your child's sleep routine can either promote or destroy the effectiveness of his own healthy immune system. Rest restores the body's strength and increases its ability to combat infections and diseases. If your child, therefore, enjoys a regular, happy, healthy sleep routine, they are less likely to fall prey to these illness-carrying adversaries as often as those children who suffer from consistent sleep deprivation.

As we have already learned, sleep plays an important role in helping to keep your child's body in optimum good health. However, sleep alone does not protect us against harmful viruses and illnesses. It is the quantity and quality of sleep that directly influences our ability to fight these infections.

The Link Between Sleep Deprivation and Overeating

Every parent is sure to be able to identify having experienced the almost desperate craving for something sweet or perhaps a tall, hot coffee on days when you feel exhausted. Sleep deprivation is believed to be one of the major causes of the development of overeating in children. When children fail to enjoy sufficient restful sleep, ghrelin, the appetite hormone, is released in the brain in increased quantities. The release of ghrelin brings about a rise in the fatty constituent (endocannabinoids) in the child's blood, increasing the desire for high-calorie foods. The sleep-deprived child often develops a yearning for foods with increased percentages of sugar and carbohydrates which offer a short-term solution to feelings of exhaustion. By continually eating foods in the high carbohydrate category, they stimulate the appetite to demand more of the same. Gradually, and almost imperceptibly in his quest for more energy, the child begins to gain unwanted weight.

Children who enjoy a healthy, happy sleep routine on the other hand, seldom experience this desire for such high carbohydrate meals because their brain and body, as well as their appetite, are already well-regulated.

The importance of instilling good, healthy, consistent sleep routines in your child ensures the creation of a firm foundation for future, successful restful sleep.

The Stages of Sleep

Sleep should not be viewed as a luxury but rather as a basic, essential part of life. In order for your child's brain to work at its optimum level, it requires a specific number of hours of uninterrupted sleep. During periods of rest, it is believed the brain sorts through all the information your child has learned and absorbed from their daily experiences and stores this as memories which can be accessed at a later stage. The brain also uses hormones released during sleep to regulate your child's moods and energy levels as well as directly influence their mental capacity and ability to learn.

It stands to reason that a child who is consistently sleep-deprived loses their chance of academic, social, and emotional success due to being tired, listless, uninterested, and probably cranky and argumentative too.

How Sleep Works

Understanding how the child's sleep patterns work and the optimal amount of sleep they require will assist the parent in choosing the correct sleep routine pattern for her child. A single, normal healthy night's sleep pattern is divided into four sleep stages lasting sixty to ninety minutes. These sleep stages are experienced by adults and children alike and each plays a vital role in the overall merit of a good night's sleep.

Sleep Stage One

Sleep Stage One is characterized by drowsiness and a sense of relaxation as alpha and beta waves are generated in the brain. This first sleep stage is described as a Non-Rapid Eye Movement (NREM) stage. Although they may appear to already be asleep, at this point, your child is actually on the brink between wakefulness and sleep. It is important to try not to disturb your child now as they can waken easily and may then experience some difficulty in falling back into sleep.

Sleep Stage Two

During Stage Two, low-frequency Theta waves are produced in the brain, which causes the child to slip into a deeper, more relaxed sleep. Breathing and heart rate begin to slow as your child's muscles relax and become limp and their body temperature begins to drop. During this stage, your child may be subconsciously aware of sounds, smells, and some sensations, but they are not likely to readily respond as they begin to lose conscious contact with the world around them. Psychologists have monitored brain waves during the second stage of sleep and discovered brief spikes in the EEG pattern. It is believed these brief, intermittent periods of activity may possibly be in response to previous learning and the resultant storage of these memories.

Sleep Stage Three

Sleep Stage Three is referred to as the deep sleep stage. It now becomes more difficult to wake the child. The child is unresponsive to touch and temperature and will generally sleep through a thunderstorm without being disturbed. Children who have a tendency to sleepwalk or talk in their sleep will do so during this period of sleep. Although breathing is very shallow and the heart rate is extremely slow during the third sleep stage, brain activity gears up several notches. Psychologists believe the majority of high-quality learning occurs at this point.

Sleep Stage Four

The fourth and final sleep stage is marked by rapid eye movements known as REM. During this stage, the brain is as active as it is during waking hours; however, the body is "dead asleep." Physical growth and tissue and cell repair take place now as the brain is busy with body and mind restoration. Essential hormones are also regulated in order to keep the body healthy and in peak condition. Dreams are believed to occur during this stage. These are believed to be the brain's tools for making sense of memories and experiences.

It is extremely difficult to wake a child from this level of sleep, and care should be taken to do this gradually in order not to shock the child. When they finally awake, they are likely to be disoriented for a few minutes and may appear pale and glassy-eyed.

Disruption in your child's sleep pattern at this point will probably leave their brain with unfinished business, resulting in them being moody and emotional, unable to make good decisions, incapable of learning new concepts, and generally not coping with the normal demands of life.

These four stages of sleep are repeated approximately every ninety minutes throughout the night and constitute a good night's sleep.

Chapter 4: The Value of Good Sleep Routines

"I can take on the world, Mom!"

How wonderful would it be to hear your child tell you they are ready for any and all the challenges each new day may bring their way?

As parents, we can all identify with the "too-exhausted-to-cope" syndrome when everything in our life appears overwhelming. Children are just as negatively affected by the lack of a good rest and may become mutinous and unsociable.

We have all experienced that comfortable, all-encompassing good feeling that comes from a restful night, and we can acknowledge a good night's sleep positively enhances all aspects of our life. Children who are fortunate enough to enjoy a good, consistent sleep routine are generally happy, focused, and filled with energy. They start each day with an enthusiastic outlook. They look forward to mastering new skills and eagerly accept challenges. These children are more capable of readily capable of absorbing facts and details and recalling this important information at a later date.

As many parents are aware, habits become a way of life. The importance of starting successful, positive habit training when your child is still in the infant stage cannot be overestimated. Preparing children as early as possible to develop the propensity to unwind and to anticipate enjoying sleeping at the end of each day will pay huge dividends in the long run for both the children and their parents. The life-long benefits of consistent periods of deep, restful sleep are the overall improvements in your child's physical, intellectual, and emotional health. This will also ensure a continued positive effect on your child's improved stamina and may possibly lead to extending their life expectancy.

Ways to Encourage Healthy Sleep Habits

The importance of implementation and maintenance of consistent sleep routines cannot be overemphasized. Parents should strive for training effective sleep routines in a calm and confident manner. The establishment of a consistent quiet period at the end of each day will be beneficial to training their child for a happy, healthy sleep routine. In order for the process to be successful, a number of simple steps should be diligently followed. These will include being aware of and understanding your child's individual personality and preferences. This is not to say that the child will dictate when, where, or how they will participate in the sleep routine. Knowledge of the child's needs, expectations, fears, age, and level of development will give the parents some valuable insight into how best to proceed with establishing a good consistent sleep routine to best suit their child.

The Peaceful, Contented Child

Living with a peaceful, contented child begins with you, the parent. Shocked though you may feel by this statement, it is true. Every parent is aware of how much happier they feel when they have a clear job description at work and how much better they cope with their workload after a good night's rest. Your child is no exception. So, to begin with, allow your child to witness your happy anticipation for a good snooze and your positive attitude the following morning when you wake well-rested. When consistent sleep routines are in place in your home, every family member will reap the benefits by the bucket load. As has already been stated, children who enjoy sufficient, restful sleep are happier, more content, and they cope better with everyday challenges. Sleep re-energizes your child's body and mind, filling them with a sense of well-being. This positive outlook on life ensures they will be more amenable to new ideas and will be more likely to look forward to the prospect of participating with enthusiasm in all aspects of their daily routine both at home and at school. Consequently, you too will be in a more positive space because there are fewer if any tantrums and tears.

The Importance of Academic Success

Every child is born with unlimited potential to grow and learn. As your young children actively explore their environment, they learn valuable information all of which, as previously reported, is collected and stored in their brain. The well-rested child has been proven to be more successful in accessing as well as retrieving this information and implementing it in order to facilitate better learning opportunities.

Sleep-deprived children, on the other hand, usually experience difficulty functioning adequately during the day because they suffer from brain exhaustion. These children often miss out as it were, and they fail to attain their full growth and learning potential because they are always too tired to become actively involved in learning and in living their life.

The long-term value of healthy sleep habits cannot be underestimated for the important role they play in your child's academic success. As previously stated, well-rested children are usually more enthusiastic about learning new skills and information because their brains and bodies are more receptive. Academic success is more easily attained when your child has the ability to focus in class and absorb and recall new information. Life, therefore, becomes more interesting and exciting for these children who have well-developed sleep routines as opposed to those who are not as fortunate to enjoy regular periods of deep, restful sleep.

During restful, uninterrupted sleep, your child's short-term memories and skills are stored in a long-term memory format, which makes for quick and easy recall when required. These improved memory skills coupled with your child's healthy sleep routine accords them the edge over many of their peers in both an academic and a social context. They will have the ability to pay attention in the classroom and subsequently increase their performance by attaining higher grades as well as enjoying affable relationships.

Studies have shown that less fortunate children on the other end of the sleep spectrum who suffer from exhaustion are often more prone to being forgetful and disorganized and are generally academically less competent.

These tired children doubtlessly struggle to remain focused for adequate periods and may, therefore, be unable to adequately absorb and assimilate new information. They are all too often the underachievers who end up dropping out of the education system as soon as they can.

Improved Creativity

As previously stated, a good sleep routine has many enormous benefits for all aspects of your child's life. Sufficient REM sleep is required for the development of your child's creativity. Sleep is not only good for your children's bodies but for the optimum functioning of their brains as well.

There is increasing evidence that sleep has a beneficial effect on our brain's ability to "join-the-dots," in a manner of speaking. During periods of deep REM sleep (see Chapter 3 for more information on the Stages of Sleep), the brain is sufficiently relaxed and able to focus on developing problem memory, solving skills, and creative ideas. When this happens, the well-rested brain is fully geared-up and capable of recognizing specific patterns as well as making sense out of a collection of unrelated data. These activities develop into problem-solving skills, beneficial to your child for decoding mathematics and scientific problems and discovering creative solutions. Children who develop these decoding skills enjoy an enhanced ability to solve puzzles and take on complicated academic and mental challenges. These children often display a better understanding of new concepts, are quicker to master new skills, and generally approach new ventures with enthusiasm.

The Link Between Sleep and Your Child's IQ

Many people believe that during sleep their body and brain are in what could be termed 'a non-functioning' state. On the contrary, however, when we sleep our body may be resting while our brain is functioning at full force. During non-rapid eye movement sleep, the brain releases short streams of energy. These energy jets were recorded on an EEG and were labeled "sleep spindles." These spindles were initially believed to represent IQ performance. More recently, these sleep spindles have been linked to periods of good, quality deep sleep. There may in fact be a definitive between children's improved IQ and the quality of sleep they enjoy. In a study involving the Rubik's cube (IQ Test Experts, n.d.), Dr. Lewis Terman discovered a single common thread in the 3,000 children tested. All those who indicated a higher IQ had structured, routine bedtimes and enjoyed a good, deep, restful sleep. It may, therefore, be possible that the greater the number of energy streams released by the brain during deep, restful sleep, the higher the IQ of the child involved. Dr. Terman recommends parents who wish to improve their children's IQ, should encourage healthy sleep routines from babyhood. Dr. Terman indicates that every hour of lost sleep your child experiences, translates to a temporary loss of one IQ point.

A further study by Fang et al. published in the *Journal of Cognitive Neuroscience*, (as cited by Thompson & Fogel, 2019) measured the quality of the sleep of the participants in the study and compared this to the characteristics of the sleep spindles. The results indicate a definite link between the spindle length and high-reasoning ability.

The adage "children who sleep better, live better" is true. Sufficient good quality sleep improves the child's ability to retain, process, and retrieve important information, and they are often more focused at school and academically smarter. They are generally more enthusiastic and successful in tackling new physical, emotional, and cognitive challenges. This results in these children doing well at school, displaying a higher IQ, and taking home better grades than their peers who have limited periods of rest and poor-quality sleep.

Chapter 5: The Causes of Sleep Problems

Because sleep is a personal process and the amount required to function at an optimum level is determined by the individual's need for sleep, it may become challenging to a parent to correctly identify the child's bedtime behavior pattern as a potential challenge to an established good sleep routine.

Good sleep routines should become a major priority for parents and their children because of their busy lifestyles and the external pressures and stresses with which they are bombarded on a daily basis. Unless parents consciously decide they need to make enough time for sleep, then it is just never going to happen.

Exaggerated, irregular sleeping patterns can be caused by a wide variety of factors that negatively impact the body's natural sleep-wake cycles, which results in these normal cycles going out of sync. If these disruptions continue for a long period, a no-sleep pattern known as insomnia begins to develop.

Consistent sleep loss or a disturbed sleep pattern often leaves children exhausted and incapable of functioning optimally during the day. Being constantly tired, the child has a marked decrease in their perceptual and cognitive functions that can lead to frequent, unnecessary accidents and injuries both at home and at school.

A lack of understanding by both parents and children of the importance of good, healthy sleep routines results in this very important aspect of life often being overlooked. In some cases, parents themselves are just too tired to argue with their willful child and succumb quickly to the child's unrealistic demands to stay up later than necessary.

The effects of interrupted or lack of sleep can have long-lasting negative implications for your child as well as your family.

Sleeping Problems - Young Children

Even with consistent sleep routines in place and despite a parent's best-laid plans, children between the ages of five and twenty-four months may suffer from sleep deprivation due to one or more of the following:

Physical Discomfort

Temperature

Regulating the temperature in your child's room is an important aspect to consider and one that will affect their quality and duration of sleep. Always ensure your baby is not in a draft and that they have sufficient bed covers. However, don't smother them! Most babies kick off their bedding and may end up wailing because they are cold. A good rule of thumb is to dress your baby suitably for the season and where possible, adjust the room temperature to a comfortable, lukewarm level. Temperature is a personal preference. What is considered a comfortable temperature in one family may either be too hot or too cold for another.

Wet diapers

Many children wake at night from the discomfort caused by a wet or leaky diaper. Try to ensure your baby has a diaper change before bedtime and again, if necessary, before the nighttime feed. Reduce the amount of fluid you give your child during the latter part of the day. In some cases, you may need to invest in nighttime diapers specially designed to contain increased amounts of moisture.

Lost pacifier

Babies develop their sucking reflex soon after birth as a way of ensuring they can breastfeed. Those infants unable to be fed by their mothers are often given a pacifier. Pacifiers are generally used to help a baby to settle at sleep time. Not all children need a pacifier. Some parents prefer not to encourage their children to become dependent on one. For various reasons, allowing your child to use a pacifier is once again a personal choice. There is some evidence of the harm that long-term use of a pacifier can cause to the proper development and growth of your child's teeth, resulting in dental deformities. Pacifiers that are not hygienically maintained can transfer a multitude of bacteria into the child's mouth. In some cases, children develop an allergy to the latex on the pacifier.

In the event of your child making use of a pacifier, they may wake due to the pacifier falling out of their mouth while they sleep. Intervention here should be quick and quiet. Replace the pacifier in your baby's mouth and return to your bed.

Crazy sleep positions

Co-sleeping with your baby can be a most gratifying or a very uncomfortable experience. This is a very personal choice which has certain advantages as well as drawbacks. If you would like to enjoy quiet, peaceful sleep then you may want to rethink co-sleeping with your baby.

Babies and toddlers move around a lot at night while they are asleep. This may be due to brain functions encouraging the child to practice what they learned during the day, such as rolling, crawling, or even standing. Often these nighttime actions are subliminal. The child follows the brain's impulses and is not actually aware of consciously moving. The results of these nighttime escapades can result in the child finally coming to rest in their cot in an awkward position.

Older children may physically fall out of bed, and some even sleepwalk and end up curled up asleep in another area in the room. When nighttime "rock-n-roll" routines cause sufficient discomfort and wake the child, gentle reassurance from the parent will usually be sufficient to get the child back on track and asleep. Parents should ensure the child is well supported in their cot or bed. For older children who sleepwalk, the addition of removable side railings to the bed or cot may help to keep the child from falling out of bed at night.

Teething challenges

Cutting teeth can cause your child to suffer from disruptive sleep. Most adults can identify with having experienced tooth pain at some point in their lifetime and know that it is no laughing matter. For some babies, this is a no-pain-no-stress matter, while for others, the debut of each new tooth is a major, painful milestone. Suitable soothing tooth and gum gels available from a reputable clinic or drugstore may do the trick of easing your child's discomfort. The child may, however, prefer to gnaw on a recommended teething device. Again, parental intervention should be kept to a minimum without fussing and undue demonstrations of emotion.

If your child wakes due to suspected teething issues, ensure you are well prepared to either face a long, sleepless night or apply some soothing gel to the affected area. It's at times such as these you may need to seek medical assistance or speak to your local clinic for advice.

Illness

In some cases, a child may suffer from disruptive sleep because they are ill. A sudden fever, frightening for any parent to witness, can wake your child and leave you panicked and stressed. If your child presents with a high fever, act swiftly. The sleep routine plans can be placed on hold for another night. The important task is to bring the child's temperature down as quickly as possible to avoid the onset of febrile convulsions. These seizures, quite terrifying to witness, usually occur in very young children as a result of an infection of some kind.

In older children, illness can present itself in the form of a sore throat, infected tonsils, abdominal pain, earache, toothache, or a multitude of other pains or rashes.

It is every parent's duty and responsibility to take care of their ill child as quickly and efficiently as possible. Remain calm and act in a sympathetic manner. Once the crisis is over, parents can resume their efforts to teach their child a good sleep routine.

Hunger and thirst

Hunger or excessive thirst can sometimes be a genuine reason for a fussy baby and the onset of a sleepless night. Newborn babies may demand to be fed almost 'around-the- clock' while for older babies up to twelve months the feeding routine usually drops from two to one feed per night. Use the nighttime feeding as an opportunity to change your baby's diaper before you feed. The secret to getting this done as quickly as possible is not to encourage your baby into believing these nighttime visits are for play and conversation. Keep everything from lighting, talking, and even rocking to a minimum. Deal with the essentials in a calm and quiet manner then put your child back into their bed and say good night.

Sleeping arrangements

Some discussion on parents co-sleeping with their child has already been mentioned under the heading Crazy Sleep Positions. There is evidence of children experiencing sleep deprivation where one or more siblings share the same bed. Too much restless movement, loss of bed covers, and lack of adequate space to lie in can have a hugely detrimental effect on the child's quality of sleep.

Emotional Discomfort

There are a number of factors that can adversely affect your child's emotional state. Some children are calmer and more laid-back than others. These children are seldom concerned about the issues that may worry other youngsters. For example, the normal house noises discernable at night do not usually bother these children who are also not disturbed by light or movement. There are many children, however, for whom the dark and nighttime hold many fears.

Fear of Excessive Noise

It is advisable to encourage your child to sleep under normal family conditions where siblings may still be up and chatting, and the muted sounds of the television or music can be heard. The child who becomes used to these household sounds may, in fact, find them soothingly familiar, and they often lull them to sleep.

There may, however, be times when sudden, unexpected, excessively loud noises such as the crash of a summer thunderstorm shock the child awake. Try not to overreact yourself, as this will surely have a detrimental effect on your child. In these instances, gentle reassurance and perhaps a night light may be sufficient to encourage the child to fall back to sleep.

Separation anxiety

Just when you thought the going was good, and your child's sleep routine was all sorted, suddenly the pattern goes haywire, and you have to start from scratch to establish a new routine. Some children experience sudden periods of extreme anxiety when they are unable to see or hear their parents. These incidents of fear-filled wailing can be most disconcerting and worrying.

Your young child may suddenly become anxious and think you have "gone missing." This is a very real problem for your child and may happen during the day or night. It is generally easier to resolve the child's anxiety in the daytime by playing peek-a-boo games or hide-and-seek. At night, however, things take a far more sinister turn when your child wakes suddenly, bewildered and anxious, and experiences a full-on panic attack.

Children, as they grow older, may also begin to develop a fear of the dark. This is a common challenge faced by many parents and usually easily resolved by placing a dim night light in the child's room. A possible solution to this challenge is to offer immediate solace, reassuring your child of your presence. Do not, however, fall into the trap of making these 'call-outs' into social, fun sessions. Keep to the routine of a calming cuddle and then lay the child back in their bed and say goodnight. This course of action isn't always as easy as it appears. The guilt that begins to set in can create huge emotional turmoil in most parents' hearts. Stay strong and consistent, parents!

Sleep Problems in Older Children

Older children between the ages of three and twelve years become very aware of changes in their environment. They are also more sensitive to nuances in adult behavior which can negatively impact their feelings of security and safety. Reassure your child of your continued presence and willingness to protect them from all harm. In cases where a divorce is imminent or already in progress, reassure your child of your devotion and commitment to them. You may require the advice and support of a professional to help you and your child work through the emotional turmoil that comes with a breakdown in family relationships. Try to maintain as many of the normal routines in the household in order to retain some sort of sense of security. The sleep routine, which may fall by the wayside for a period of time, should be reinforced as soon as possible.

Night Terrors

Preschool children are not yet fully aware of reality and will often be caught up mentally and emotionally in a world of make-believe. Sometimes these childhood fantasies are harmless and full of excitement and happiness. Others, however, can encourage your preschool child's imagination to run riot, resulting in nightmares and terrors that negatively impact your child's sleep routine and may in some cases prohibit peaceful sleep for long periods. In an attempt to avoid these night terrors, it is important for parents to monitor suitable television programs, games, movies, and stories for this age group.

Normal Childhood Fears and Anxiety

For many children in this age group, it is considered normal to suffer from a fear of the dark or strange nighttime noises. Dim light or suitable, soft music may help the child overcome these fears. A number of other possible fears or phobias that can manifest at nighttime may include for example the 'monster' under the bed or behind the door, a branch tapping against a windowpane, or the sound of the refrigerator switching on and off. Each of these fears is very real for your child, so don't belittle them or tease them about this. During the daytime, talk to your child about fear and try to elicit the source. Find creative ways to support their sense of safety and security by helping them overcome their fears. Sometimes a 'cuddle buddy' in the form of a soft toy may help the child feel more secure. Sleep routine often takes a hard knock in instances of nighttime fear. Try to reinforce the sleep routine as soon as possible.

Excessive Competition

Older children often experience a very real fear of excessive competition in the home or at school. These fears can create feelings of inadequacy and anxiety that may derail not only your child's sleeping pattern but their entire sense of well-being. The result of fear of competition can be a drop in school grades, a negative change in attitude at home, or may manifest as a loss of self-confidence and the development of low self-esteem. The child may lose interest in social activities and become a bench sitter during activities rather than a participant. Again, the importance of a good, healthy sleep routine cannot be sufficiently overemphasized. Parents should get the ball rolling again as soon as possible and reinstate the sleep time routine.

Cyber or Social Media Bullying

Older children may become the victims of cyber or social media bullying which will most certainly cause anxiety and sleep disruption. Many children find it difficult to disclose bullying for fear of negative repercussions. Parents should be on the lookout for any sudden changes in their child's behavior. These may be evident in sudden bouts of unexplained anger or tears. Some children who were previously socially active may become withdrawn and reclusive. The challenge for parents is identifying their child's fear and addressing it as soon as possible. By being a sympathetic, hands-on parent, you may be able to encourage your child to talk about these fears and give you the chance to assist them in dealing with them. In many instances, however, children struggling with these fears require professional advice and support.

Depression and Eating Disorders

Depression is classed as a behavioral disorder and has become a very real problem for modern children. Depression can have its roots in a multitude of circumstances. It can develop as a result of the sudden death of a family member or a beloved pet. The ever-increasing divorce rate can have a long-term negative effect on the child's emotional state. Domestic violence in the home or being placed in foster care may leave the child in an emotional turmoil with feelings of desolation and abandonment. In each of these instances, the child will suffer from sleep deprivation and a lack of a good sleep routine.

Sleep deprivation also sabotages the manufacture of ghrelin and leptin, which are hormones that regulate feelings of hunger and maintain sugar levels in the blood. These hormones are usually produced during periods of restful, relaxed sleep. A decrease in the production of these hormones in children as a result of sleep disorders encourages them to turn to food for solace and comfort. In many cases, these children develop eating disorders which in turn lead to bulimia nervosa, anorexia nervosa, or obesity.

So, it's back to emphasizing the vital importance of healthy sleep routines for children and indeed for every member of the family.

Chapter 6: Sleep Deprivation - The Negative Impact

Children who experience difficulty sleeping due to the lack of consistent, good routines often become overtired and too wired to fall asleep. These children will sometimes avoid bedtime, making any number of excuses to stay up later than necessary. The later they stay up, the crankier they are and the more desperate the parents become. This sort of behavior can escalate into a destructive spiral in which the entire family becomes victims of the "chase-your-tail" scenario.

Social and Emotional Bonds

Good social skills often diminish with a lack of sleep. The child with a poor sleep routine is often cranky, overtired, and too emotional to see reason. This behavior pattern escalates and is likely to affect the entire family unit, impacting negatively on all areas of each member's life. Daily tasks begin to appear insurmountable for the sleep-deprived child whose brain becomes too tired to absorb new information. This awareness of failure may lead to a defeatist attitude, and the child may then begin to experience a sense of rejection and develop low self-esteem.

Tired children lack the energy to socialize. They often prefer to remain isolated or hover on the periphery of a social group. When these sleep-deprived children are confronted with social conflict issues, they will either fight or flee. They lack the emotional maturity and skills to deal adequately with any conflict. These children may not have many friends and those they choose often display similar patterns of behavior to their own.

Well-rested children usually demonstrate dependable characteristics and develop improved self-esteem. They cope better with social challenges and feel sufficiently validated through their acceptance into their social circle. They demonstrate a calm, happy attitude and are less likely to become involved in social or emotional squabbles which may in some instances, lead to physical skirmishes. They often exhibit improved perceptual and intellectual skills which empower them to weigh potentially dangerous situations with wisdom, rather than act in an irrational emotional manner as do those children who experience insufficient sleep.

Good sleeping patterns assist in the production of positive endorphins. These hormones, known fondly as "happy hormones," are released in the child's brain during periods of restful sleep. Their job is to help the child remain cheerful and calm. Calm children are more manageable and cooperative both individually and in group situations. It makes sense then that such children are likely to have a more positive outlook at school and their success in the classroom is almost guaranteed.

Inappropriate Behavior Escalates

Every parent has at some point in their parenting career experienced feelings of exasperation or irritation and may display limited patience after several nights of a disturbed night of sleep.

Imagine how much worse these feelings are for a child who has neither the resources nor the maturity to cope in this situation, beyond of course, losing his cool.

Parents should be aware of the indication of attention problems, hyperactivity, bullying and aggressive behavior, as well as mood swings and anxiety, are negative behaviors being attributed to children with depleted sleep patterns. A recent study found that higher cognitive functions including abstract thinking, verbal creativity, and verbal reasoning become impaired in children between the ages of 10 and 14 years after just a single night of limited sleep.

The Impact on Self-Esteem

Tired children usually don't feel at peace with themselves or the world. They are often miserable because their brains are too exhausted to function adequately. A sleep-deprived brain is incapable of making sense of information in a quick and effective manner. Simple activities may appear impossible to a sleep-deprived child, and these tasks become too burdensome to manage. The tired child fears failure, which in turn leads to feelings of insecurity. They may become moody and withdrawn, refusing to participate in activities at home and at school. In some instances, these children may thrive on the increased attention their action creates and may make use of this attention to escalate their negative behavior patterns.

New situations and changes are often viewed with trepidation by children with poor sleep routines. Children who do not enjoy sufficient sleep are likely to be less willing to accept change. They are often fearful of stepping into new situations because many of these sleep-deprived children suffer from excess cortisol in the brain. Cortisol is a stress-release hormone released during wakefulness. Children with an excess of this hormone are unable to relax and fall asleep. Their bodies are in a constant state of anxiety which can over time lead to serious illnesses including type 2 diabetes and heart disease as well as weight gain challenges culminating in obesity.

Substandard Academic Achievement

It stands to reason tired children cannot function well in the academic field. Their grades often drop due to their inability to stay focused in the classroom and they are often slow to recall information. The negative impact their lack of academic progress has on these children's self-esteem can be devastating. Continued lack of rest or disrupted sleep escalates into a never-ending cyclic stress scenario. According to Sumi Rose from the Acharya Institute of Health Science, Bangalore, (Research Gate, n.d.), insufficient sleep, which is a basic biological necessity for life, has a serious negative impact on academic success. Cognitive functions including memory, concentration, and attention are compromised by lack of sufficient sleep. This results in a decline in overall academic performance as the brain loses its ability to function optimally and becomes foggy from lack of sleep.

It becomes vitally important for the parents to take control and introduce their child to good sleep routines as early as possible. Teaching your child the important value of healthy sleep habits will have long-term beneficial results for your child's overall health and well-being.

Attention-Deficit

Scientists believe there is a direct link between children suffering from learning difficulties and attention deficit challenges and irregular sleeping patterns. Despite this link between sleep deprivation and attention-deficit not yet having been proven, tired children are known to sometimes become hyperactive because they enter and remain in an overtired state due to the excessive production of adrenalin. Heart ailments and stress-related diseases, which may develop as a direct result of sleep deprivation, are becoming more prevalent in children during this decade.

Psychosomatic Illnesses

When children experience poor or interrupted sleep routines and may be too tired to face each day, they can unconsciously develop symptoms of a health disorder without any tangible medical proof of the source for the physical disease. Although there is a direct correlation between exhaustion and psychosomatic illness, which include eczema, psoriasis, high blood pressure, ulcers, and heart disease (Henderson, 2016), children who suffer from this disorder may, although not in every instance, be the victims of interrupted sleep. They may resort to complaining about head or stomach aches in order to avoid attending class or in an attempt to draw attention away from their plight of lack of sleep.

Inadequate Physical Growth and Sleeplessness

Holly McGurgan and Jessica Kania (2018) suggest growth delays can be attributed to a number of factors including insufficient growth hormone (GH) or a condition known as hypothyroidism, which is due to an underactive thyroid. Some children are naturally shorter than their peers simply because of their genetic composition. Certain types of anemia and diseases of the heart, lungs, or kidneys can also be responsible for significant delays in a child's growth. Poor nutrition and living conditions are also important considerations. However, researchers believe there may be a connection between delayed growth and a consistent lack of good quality sleep. As previously noted, stress is often associated with poor sleep routines.

Irregular sleep minimizes growth spurts which are believed to occur during periods of peaceful rest. The lack of good sleep routines may result in stunted physical, mental, emotional, and academic development. If your child wakes up feeling tired and grumpy, the chances are they are not getting sufficient sleep.

Immune System

As many as one in three children can be identified as a sleep-deprived sufferer. The reasons for their plight are often multifaceted and difficult to pinpoint. However, stress is definitely an important factor. Lack of good routines, violence in the home, poor social choices, drug addiction, and the continued use of electronic devices added to the mix creates a powerfully dangerous scenario for the risks of type 2 diabetes, heart disease, and obesity for children suffering from sleep deprivation. These illnesses are often carried into adulthood, and when high blood pressure is then added to the list, life expectancy rapidly decreases.

The immune system plays a vital role in helping to protect the body against infections and illnesses. Studies done at Vanderbilt University School of Medicine indicate a definite link between sleep disorders and a compromised immune system (Wu & Van Kaer, 2011) as the percentage of T-cells, responsible for protection against illness, decrease when a child suffers from sleep deprivation.

Cytokines that encourage inflammation then begin to increase and break down the body's safeguard barriers. The conclusion he draws is that sleep loss compromises the child's immune system and improves their chance of contracting diseases and becoming ill. The long-term effects of sleep loss negatively impact personal health to such an extent that their situation can develop into a war between life and death.

Overall Poor Performance

When children miss out on sufficient good REM sleep, they become less likely to cope with daily challenging tasks. For these sleep-deprived children, their social skills are often the first to disintegrate because they are unable to positively identify the important social and emotional clues used daily for successful communication.

The second set of skills to take a dive includes mental and academic skills such as memory, computing, and language ability.

When the brain suffers from sleep deprivation, it tries to compensate by forcing the child to sleep lightly over a shorter period of time. The starvation of REM sleep makes concentration and multitasking almost impossible for your child. They may become easily confused, lose the thread of instructions, and be unable to figure out the answers to basic questions.

Good, healthy sleep routines for all children are vital in order for them to receive sufficient, deep, relaxing rest.

Chapter 7: Signs of Sleep Deprivation

Parents who have not instituted a good sleep routine for their children may be doing them a serious disservice. According to Gerber (2014), on the subject of sleep deprivation, the growing number of children suffering from sleep deprivation is reaching alarming proportions.

Unfortunately, many parents survive each day on minimum sleep. This pattern of behavior now appears to be affecting their children. Gerber suggests the statistics of sleep-deprived humans have become "a public health epidemic." Gerber's article focuses on the effect sleep deprivation has on children between the ages of five and eighteen years. There is reported evidence that children in this category display a higher percentage of eating disorders, depression, mood swings, aggressive behavior, impulse control issues, and poor academic achievement (Gerber, 2014).

Although it is never too late to teach their children the value of getting sufficient rest, some parents may miss the signs of sleep deprivation in their child.

Sleep Disorders

Although sleep disorders are more prevalent now than ever before, indications that children are suffering from lack of sleep are sometimes dismissed as bad behavior. If your children regularly displays more than three of these symptoms, they are likely to be suffering the effects of sleep deprivation, and it may be time to re-evaluate their sleeping routine in order to assist them.

Slow to Wake

Is your child slow to wake each morning and reluctant to get out of bed? Everyone experiences mornings when their bed seems to be the best place to spend the day, especially when the weather turns unexpectedly chilly. Aside from the 'sleepy teen' syndrome, where children may be out later at night at social events, being reluctant to get out of bed each morning may not be unusual. However, children who go to bed at a reasonable time and who wake late on a daily basis may not have enjoyed sufficient restful sleep. These children may be glassy-eyed, display dark circles beneath their eyes, and want to nap frequently throughout the day.

Short Attention Span and Lack of Focus

Does your child display a noticeably short attention span and are they unable to recall information and participate in simple conversations? Many children lose interest at some point in listening to their parents or following a conversation that may mean little to them. However, if your child struggles to remember basic information about school sport-fixtures for instance or dates and times of regular appointments, forgets to take the correct sports kit or an item of clothing, and is unable to focus when spoken to, they may be suffering from sleep deprivation. It is a proven fact that children with poor attention experience difficulties in remaining focused at school.

Hyperactivity and Disruptive Behavior

Does your child display hyperactive and unacceptably disruptive behavior? Sleep deprivation may be the underlying cause. Lack of good, restful sleep robs the child of normal mental impulses that govern behavior. As previously mentioned, due to intermittent or disturbed sleep patterns, insufficient endorphins (happy hormones) are produced. In addition, excess production of adrenalin keeps the body in a constant hyperactive state. When a child suffers from a consistent lack of good restful sleep, they may appear to turn into the proverbial "monster" because they have reached a state of total exhaustion.

Lacks Motivation

It is unrealistic for parents to expect their children to live in a constantly motivated state. Every busy child requires adequate rest in order to function at their best. If your child has been a successful student who suddenly shows a decreased interest and motivation in learning and attending school, they may be in need of a few really good, undisturbed nights' sleep. However, if their usually positive and enthusiastic attitude to attending school drops off markedly, and they become disinterested in learning, their sleep routine may require some tweaking in order for them to get back on track.

Clumsy Behavior

Although there may be other medical reasons why children fall and injure themselves more often, the parent's first port-of-call should be to examine the child's sleeping pattern. According to the research done by Gerber (2014), children who suffer from consistent sleep deprivation become too tired to focus. They lack good coordination, appear clumsy, and may become accident-prone.

Frequent Illness

Sleep-deprived children often suffer from unexplained colds and infections due to a compromised immune system that takes a beating when the child suffers from a lack of good quality sleep. Good sleep, in regular doses as we now know, is a natural requirement for our bodies and minds to work at their best.

According to Gerber (2014), there is a definite correlation between regular sleep patterns and the body's ability to adequately repair damaged cells and tissues.

In instances where a lack of sleep prevails, these essential repairs are not completed, leaving the body vulnerable to further attacks from viruses and germs. Among the illnesses that are more prevalent due to sleep deprivation are:

Epstein-Barr Virus

This virus causes extreme tiredness, and it becomes difficult for sufferers to cope with the demands of a normal daily life. It may have an increased effect on sleep-deprived children who are already compromised and more vulnerable to contracting viral infections than those who enjoy sufficient shut-eye.

Asthma

Poorly controlled illnesses such as asthma leave the child exhausted due to a severe lack of oxygen. This condition is exacerbated by a lack of sleep. Children suffering from asthma are generally unable to participate in strenuous activities without added medical support.

Anemia

The blood carries oxygen to all areas of the body. When the percentage of red blood cells drops due to an infection or illness, the amount of oxygen circulating in the blood decreases exponentially. This usually results in extreme fatigue and a severe lack of energy. Children suffering from anemia are usually very pale and listless. They prefer to participate in non-strenuous activities and will more than likely choose to stay indoors.

Hypothyroidism

This illness, which is the result of a reduction in the release of the thyroxine hormone that helps to regulate metabolism, often causes extreme fatigue and moodiness. There is a definable link between hypothyroidism and lack of sleep, and it may develop as a result of stress due to interrupted sleep.

Heart Problems

Although generally rare, heart illness can lead to chronic exhaustion due to the inability of the heart to pump sufficient oxygen-carrying blood to all the organs. Gerber (2014) indicates an increase in the number of children suffering from heart conditions. Although some of these are in fact physiological in nature, others can be attributed to the stress of poor sleep routines and the lack of good, quality sleep.

Cancer

This illness is becoming more common in children and may be a result of lifestyle, poor eating habits, or pollution. Continued sleeplessness can be a contributing factor.

Constant Yawning

Yawning is a common external sign of being tired. By yawning, the body attempts to increase the flow of oxygen to the lungs, thus supplying the brain and other organs with this life-giving air.

Children who yawn excessively are more than likely suffering from sleep deprivation. These children may often nod off in the car or in front of the television. They can, however, also fall asleep in class or during a period of homework.

Parents should be on the lookout for these behavior traits as they signal the need for immediate adult intervention and the reestablishment of a good sleep routine.

Aggressive Behavior

Children who suffer from sleep deprivation often display aggressive behavior and may even throw temper tantrums that are not considered age appropriate. This is a behavior characteristic is sometimes expected of two-year-olds so if older children are resorting to unusual or unexpected aggressive behavior, parents should examine their children's sleep routine.

Children who have poor sleep routines may often exhibit a low tolerance for frustration. They are unable to complete tasks and lose interest halfway through a project. They are often antisocial and find interacting with others exhausting.

Bed-Wetting

If all other medical and physiological avenues have first been explored and come up with negative results, a sudden onset of bedwetting can signal your child is overtired and not getting enough good quality rest. Although bedwetting can be the result of anxiety or fear, consistent, restful sleep routines may be the solution to the problem.

Snoring

Most adults and children snore at some point during their sleep. However, if these episodes reach a stage where normal breathing becomes sufficiently disrupted to wake the child from sleep, then medical intervention should be sought. Continued sleep disruption due to snoring will lead to broken sleep, resulting in insufficient rest. This can have a detrimental effect on the entire family.

Sleepwalking or Night Terrors

Some children sleepwalk at night, which can result in a restless night and a fitful sleep. Although many children who suffer from this affliction are not consciously aware of moving around in the night, once they wake up from an episode, they may have difficulty trying to get back to sleep.

Night terrors can be very disturbing for a child, as well as his parents. Fear of the dark, the shadows that appear to move at night, and perhaps even fear of the "monster" under the bed are very real fears for children who suffer from night terrors.

Sleep disruption can occur more than once a night and can be repeated night after night. This is an exhausting situation for both the child and his parents.

Restless Leg Syndrome

This behavior occurs when children involuntarily move their legs while they are lying down. There is often no detrimental effect on the individual child; however, if they share a bed, their sibling or parent will definitely be disturbed.

Chapter 8: The Dangers of Technology for Children

The vast amount of innovative technology developed specifically for children has increased dramatically over the past two decades and now accounts for one of the largest groups of technology worldwide. Children's access to mobile devices has also increased fivefold during this period, and many such devices are being used daily as teaching aids in the classroom.

The extensive growth of technology has completely changed virtually every aspect of our society. As a result, all the dimensions of our children's lives from home to school and their personal, as well as social relationships, have been impacted. And it has not stopped there. The long arm of technological influence extends not only to the choices of food available and the style of clothing children wear but dominates their music and electronic gadgetry and has caused a paradigm shift in their view of life and expectations.

The Impact of Increased Technology Use on Children

According to a recent survey of the parents of 234 children between the ages of eight and seventeen years, they indicated the daily use of technological devices (computers, tablets, video games, cell phones, and television) (Fuller, Lehman, Hicks, & Novick, 2017), especially prior to bedtime, showed a marked negative influence on the number of hours as well as the quality of sleep these children enjoyed. A definite link between the long-term use of technology and the increase in inattentive behavior was evident.

Many inventive electronic devices and tablet-based children's toys that offer innovative learning opportunities have in fact unintended negative consequences on certain areas of the child's development. With specific reference to the growth and progress of motor skills coordination, many children are experiencing delays. Intellectually, device-driven children demonstrate an inability to focus, pay attention, and recall important information. On an emotional and social level, the consistent use of electronic gadgetry has a marked negative impact on the development of the child's language skills and their ability to form friendships.

Restful sleep is fundamental to the optimal functioning of the body and mind during childhood. There is a definite link between lack of sleep in children and the development of behavioral and emotional disorders. Spending hours watching television also increases anxiety levels and negatively impacts the child's ability to fall asleep and stay asleep. Many modern children take their cell phones to bed with them where they then text or play games well into the night. This activity ensures poor sleep routines.

Poor sleep quality is believed to have a direct link to hyperactivity and attention deficit problems in children. It has been discovered that consistent, early exposure of children to television resulted in the development of attention disorders by the time these children were in middle school.

An interesting relationship between the use of technology and increased BMI indicates users, especially children, are becoming less active and more sedentary. Their body mass increases proportionally to the amount of time spent working or playing on their devices. Consequently, it appears that many children spend more time indoors than out. However, it's important to encourage children to spend some time outdoors in order to benefit from Vitamin D absorption, which in turn supports the body's natural security system in fighting off viruses.

A good period of time in the sunshine may help the body adjust to the day-night cycle. Hypothetically speaking, by remaining indoors for long periods, the child's brain may not be able to distinguish night from day. This confusion can upset the body's natural time cycle and may lead to sleep difficulties.

Other factors including the children's safety and security may also influence this trend of "Life appears better on the inside!"

Results of The Survey Into the Use of Technology

The results of the survey by Fuller et al. (2017) indicate a direct correlation between the extended use of technology devices and reduced sleep patterns in children. Continued exposure to electronic and technology use is now known to increase children's brain activity and substantially bump-up their anxiety levels. Children who watch more than two hours of television per day are more likely to suffer inattention and have difficulty recalling relevant information in an academic setting. Overuse of technology by children has a direct link to weight gain and the early onset of type 2 diabetes. In most instances, children who make consistent use of technology devices become increasingly sedentary and lose interest in participating in outdoor activities. For many of these children, the extended use of technology becomes a way of life. It is possible that the percentage of individuals suffering from obesity is, therefore, on the increase.

Aggression and negative social behavior can be attributed to the extended use of technological devices by children. The younger the child, the greater the long-term impact on their behavior and sleep routines. Children who continually make use of electronic devices tend to become less sociable and experience difficulty in communicating adequately face-to-face. These children often fail to identify social clues and struggle to develop meaningful, lasting relationships. The negative impact this has on the development of good language skills and interpersonal relationships can be far-reaching.

Children who spend a great deal of time interacting with electronic devices learn at an early age to multitask. They are bombarded by information and stimuli that keep their brain in a constant state of flux. Although these children may be smart and on-the-ball because they can quickly work through problems and facts on a superficial level, they appear to be losing the ability to focus and think creatively and critically.

Is It All Negative?

Whether or not we agree with the use of electronic devices, technology is here to stay. In many ways, it has brought humanity numerous wonderful opportunities for entertainment, socializing, teaching, and learning as well as affording us the opportunity to communicate over vast distances, quickly and effectively. Each day of our lives we make use of technology devices in one form or another, from cooking to transportation, from connecting with friends and family far and wide to ordering our shopping or clothing online.

Without technology, there would never have been space exploration nor would man have had the chance to walk on the moon.

All in all, it appears that although our children are surrounded by electronic technology devices, careful, judicial management of the use of these gadgets is essential for our overall optimum development. Instead of prohibiting the use of technology in the home, parents should take the responsibility to monitor their children's use of the devices. Parents should consider creating opportunities to enjoy family events and occasions that take all the members outdoors more often. Planning family walks, maybe camping or fishing trips, ice-skating, or just playing in the snow and creating beautiful snow angels enjoying outdoor activities. Sometimes, it is the simple, inexpensive activities that end up being the most fun.

Chapter 9: Possible Solutions to Sleep Disruption

Optimal sleep is an essential aspect for every human's well-being. According to many mental health and wellness gurus, quality sleep is a necessity, not a luxury without which we cannot enjoy a happy, healthy, and successful life.

So, how do these already exhausted parents find a suitable solution to overcoming the challenges of their sleep-deprived child? The secret to a successful sleep routine strategy is to start early and remain consistent. Once the child is in a good routine, life for the entire family unit will improve. A number of other strategies that may prove useful to get your child off to sleep are mentioned below.

Parental Control

Tracy Hogg (as cited by Timmons, 2016), suggests parents should realize they are in control of teaching their child a healthy sleep routine. By setting a good example themselves, their children will begin to understand the importance of going to bed each night at the required time.

Many parents harbor guilt about appearing as the 'ogre' in their family because they institute rules and boundaries for their children. Parents should throw the guilt out immediately and realize their child has no other way of learning the rules for life other than by the example set by the parents themselves.

Being consistent in setting up rules of any kind is the key to success. Make sure your child goes to bed at the same time every night. Maintain as rigid a time frame as is feasible for your family, so that the child knows by 7 p.m., they are expected to be in bed. This behavior will in time become a good habit that is automatically followed, thus ensuring fewer future tears and dramas at the end of the day.

Do not be tempted to offer your child food or drink just before bedtime, and ensure one of their final activities before sleeping is a visit to the bathroom. Avoid bribery and punishment when teaching your child any routine or skills as neither of these actions produces any lasting satisfactory results. Many newborns prefer to sleep on their tummies. This sleeping position, though comfortable for the baby, has been linked to Sudden Infant Death Syndrome and is therefore not recommended. Parents of newborns should, therefore, encourage the baby to sleep on their backs. Some babies resist this position and may require a little assistance to start with. A little trick that may help to get baby comfortable is to place a bolster (a long, rolled, sausage-shaped cushion) behind their back to keep them lying slightly on their side. This may offer your baby the added support they need.

Between the ages of three and six months, your baby's sleeping habits change. There may be a noticeable regression in their sleep patterns. Your baby is developing an awareness of all the new and exciting sights around them. This may result in them becoming overstimulated, which results in your baby not wanting to sleep! Sleep regression is usually a temporary phenomenon, and with patience and consistent reinforcement of the sleep routine, your baby will eventually find a balance that suits them and you.

Older children, from around six months of age, sometimes find it difficult to fall back asleep after they have woken during the night. This is a skill these children need to learn. Consistent sleep routine training will help the child develop self-soothing techniques (sucking their thumb or a pacifier), and they will fall back to sleep. This, of course, may take time so don't expect a miracle cure!

Some Ideas to Assist Your Child in Falling Asleep Quickly

Happy, stress-free babies and children usually have well-established sleep routines. These children have a distinct advantage over those who are not as fortunate to enjoy a good rest at night.

Consistency and patience are the primary keys to the successful establishment of good sleep routines. The responsibility for structuring and implementing these routines falls squarely on the shoulders of the parents. Because each child has their own individual personality and specific needs, they may take longer to unwind and relax at bedtime. Some great ideas follow that for parents to consider to support their child's easier transition to asleep.

Hand or foot reflexology/massage

Your child's little hands and feet have been extremely busy all day touching, lifting, carrying, building, walking, tiptoeing, running, and maybe even kicking. A lot of tension can develop in these busy little muscles, so why not gently massage your child's hands and feet before bedtime? Massage releases tension and creates a sense of trust and well-being that is calming to your child.

Spending quality time like this with your child doesn't have to take longer than a few minutes and will also have a positive effect on you, the parent.

Peaceful music or singing

Some children respond to the soothing sounds of relaxing music or mom's soft singing. These rhythmic sounds may help your child fall asleep more quickly and without any fuss. There is a delightful range of useful, child-friendly apps and gadgets that may assist with getting your child to readily doze off each night. Please see the sections on Apps for Children and Sleep Gadgets to Help Your Child Fall Asleep.

Rocking

Gentle rhythmic rocking movements can have a soporific effect on some children. Parents may discover this is a slam-dunk way of getting their child to sleep. This action can prove to be calming and soothing for both parent and child. Some schools of thought reckon rocking is not the best way to get your baby to sleep. They suggest rocking should, as far as possible, be restricted to the bedtime routine and should not become a demand pattern of relaxation. The choice is up to the parent!

A "cuddle buddy"

Some children find comfort in hugging and snuggling up at bedtime with a special soft toy, a fluffy blanket, a special piece of smooth textured fabric, or even an old shirt of dad's. The sense of security this brings your child may well support their need for extra comfort at night. If it works, wonderful!

It may be a good idea to offer a different "cuddle buddy" each night to avoid the child becoming fixated on just one toy. This is of particular importance should your child loses their favorite soft toy, or it has to go into the washing machine.

Bedtime stories

Older children may enjoy a bedtime story to calm them down at the end of a busy day. Not only is reading considered a valuable skill for your child's future academic success but this quality story time with their parents is also a great bonding opportunity and strengthens your child's sense of belonging and security. There are a number of really useful apps that support bedtime reading. A few of these are noted in the section Sleep Gadgets to Help Your Child Fall Asleep

Sleep Training for Successful Sleep Routines

A number of sleep training methods may be well worth considering in assisting your child in developing a happy, healthy sleep routine. Each of these methods has merits of its own, but because every child is different, it may be worthwhile for the parents to try to establish their own child's personal pattern.

Cry-it-out method of sleep training

The cry-it-out method advocates the baby should be left to cry for a substantial amount of time before the parent intervenes and offers support. There is no current empirical evidence available that this method results in children with social and emotional issues.

This method was conceived by Dr. Emmett Holt and first published in 1895 in *The Care and Feeding of Children*. It was later popularized by Dr. Richard Ferber in his book *Solve Your Child's Sleep Problems*, first published in 1985, and may not perhaps be the most popular method for training sleep routine in very young children. However, greater success may be a result of those babies around six months or older.

Although Dr. Marc Weissbluth, renowned author of *Healthy Sleep Habits, Happy Child* (as cited by Johnson, 2019b), suggests a number of different sleep methods. He advocates the cry-it-out method as being the best option. Many parents are not comfortable with this method as they believe it is too harsh for a new baby.

Maressa Brown, a contributing writer and editor at What to Expect (Brown, 2016), comments on the cry-it-out method as being useful for some babies. However, she adds that when parents are consistent in their minimum response to the "call out," the baby soon realizes his parents are not going to respond to his demands and he will eventually settle down and will learn to self-soothe. Sounds so easy, doesn't it? The challenge here is of course, that no two babies respond the same way to any sleep method offered. Often the best option for parents is to try out a number of methods, take the best ideas from each, and combine them to create your baby's personal sleep pattern.

The benefits of the cry-it-out method:
- Babies can exhibit less stress.

- Babies eventually learn to fall asleep faster.

The drawbacks of this method:
- Babies may develop a negative association with sleeping that can have a life-long effect.

- The constant crying of the child is emotionally disturbing for parents.

- Highly sensitive babies may end up choking from crying too hard or too long.

No tears method of sleep training

This method advocates a gentler approach to sleep training. Its main aim is to reduce crying and increase the child's feelings of security and well-being.

Important aspects to bear in mind with this method:
- A consistent bedtime routine is a vital component.

- Encourage your child to go to sleep when they begin to show signs of being tired.

- Children generally drop off to sleep faster.

- Keep the environment quiet and calm.

- Use consistent phrases your child will begin to identify as "bedtime routine talk."

- Reassure your baby as often as is needed.

The positive aspects of this method:
- Babies may cry less.

- Babies may settle down fairly quickly to sleep.

- This method offers the opportunity for bonding between parent and child.

The negative aspects to consider:
- Babies can become more dependent on parents for comfort.

- Babies do not develop the ability to soothe themselves.

Fading-it-out method of sleep training

This sleep training method is more popular than the cry-it-out method because it advocates sleep preparation with some tears.

Parents who choose this method, allow their child to fall asleep in their own time over a period of approximately five nights. They then start the sleep routine 15 minutes earlier for the next five consecutive nights. This pattern is repeated over a period of time until the child begins to sleep regularly at an acceptable time. Running concurrently to this method, parents may continue to use rocking, singing, or a pacifier or whatever else they find works for their baby. These added activities run the risk, however, of making baby dependent on the extra support that is being offered. Parents should remain vigilant in maintaining the routine structure. Keep your eye on the end goal: getting baby off to sleep as soon as possible!

The challenge with this method is the time factor, which may not always be feasible for parents who work a full day and who are already exhausted by the time they should be getting their baby ready for bed.

The value of this method:
- There is ample opportunity for baby-parent bonding.

- Babies generally cry less.

- With consistent patience, the reward of having the baby finally sleeping well outweighs the effort required to achieve this goal.

- Babies have opportunities to self-comfort.

- Babies feel more secure.

The negative aspects of this method:
- Time constraints may become a challenge.

- The parent must buy into this method and commit to the consist effort it requires to be successful.

- Babies can become dependent on "sleep props."

- Overanxious parents may become more stressed.
- There is no one-size-fits-all method.

And When All Else Fails?

When parents reach a point of being so exhausted they can no longer think straight or where their small person just simply refuses all efforts to settle them for the night after night, it may be time to call in the Ghostbusters! No, seriously, it may be time to seek professional help. So, where do you begin?

Child Psychology

The child psychologist may be the best professional to contact for advice and support. Your local clinic or medical practitioner's office is sure to have some information. Otherwise, your next best option will be to surf the net. Technology has its uses!

Child psychology is the study of how children grow and interact with their environment. It includes an evaluation of the child's stages of development from birth to about the age of 18 years and determines how well children cope at each level of development.

The results of these observations and studies assist the child psychologist in determining the cause of a particular detrimental change in behavior. The psychologist is then able to suggest possible solutions.

There are five main areas of interest to the Child Psychologist:

The development of the child

Included here is cognitive, emotional, social as well as physical development.

- Cognitive Development

Cognitive, also known as intellectual development, refers to the processes of learning, which include the acquisition of language and the ability to develop thought processes and problem-solving skills. These skills are of vital importance for success in the classroom.

- Emotional and Social Development

These usually go hand-in-hand and they are interdependent areas. Included here are the development of self-esteem, the ability to recognize and respond correctly to emotional signals, and the ability to interact cooperatively in a group and to display the correct reaction to specific feelings such as happiness, fear, and humor. Children who are emotionally and socially well-balanced are happier and more capable of making lasting friendships.

- Physical Development

Pertains to the physical growth of the child and includes height, mass, and general growth spurts. Gross-motor skills like walking, running, hopping, throwing, catching, stretching, bending, and crawling form an important part of physical growth. Fine- motor skills such as cutting, threading, folding paper, coloring in, and writing are also important physical skills. These skills support sports development and good hand-eye coordination.

Important Milestones

Developmental milestones are those specific levels of achievement children should automatically achieve on their path to adulthood. Each milestone indicates a specific level of development. The child psychologist uses these milestones as a way of measuring the child's performance. The child who struggles to reach each of these levels within a given time will require the correct intervention and support to help them achieve their goals.

The main areas of interest include learning difficulties, attention disorders, and hyperactivity, and emotional issues such as anxiety and depression.

Behavior

As children grow and develop, they go through different stages of behavior. These include the "terrible twos" through the stages of defiance and conflict with parents and other figures of authority. In cases where these behavior patterns escalate and children become violent, aggressive, or disruptive at home and at school, the child psychologist can step in to assist.

Child behavior is affected by a number of emotional scenarios, from divorce or a death in the family to a fall out with friends. Attention difficulties, as well as hyperactivity, are forms of deviant behavior. It becomes vital for the child psychologist to determine the root cause of the problem before any solution can be given.

Emotions

Every child experiences feelings of happiness, loneliness, fear, and anxiety. When these feelings overwhelm the child and interfere with their normal growth and development or impact negatively on their intellectual achievements, help is required.

Socialization

The ability to develop the skills to make and maintain friendships as well as communicate adequately with others and work cooperatively in a group fall into this category. Through play in early childhood, children acquire valuable social and conflict management skills.

The importance of the parents' role in the child's development

Despite the socio-economic status of the home, all children need to know they are loved and that their parents will provide for them and keep them safe.

The parents' duty to their children cannot be underestimated. Parents should be committed to stepping up for their children and taking the lead in the family. As previously stated, parents act as role models for their children.

Conclusion: Don't Give Up!

Because sleep is such an essential component of every child's life, it is vitally important for parents to encourage their little "busy-bodies" to buy into this valuable part of their daily schedule. A vast number of suggestions have been made to assist parents with the sometimes daunting task of getting their rambunctious child to sleep.

Parental Example

Parents should set the best example they can and be mindful of the fact that their children mimic their parents' actions, body language, and vocabulary. The environment becomes an important factor for sleepless children when there is excessive noise, light, movement, or room temperature that disturbs their sleep routine. The wailing of a new baby in the household can have a serious negative impact on a sibling's quality of sleep.

Sleep Routines

One of the most valuable routines parents can bestow on their child is that of a good, healthy sleep pattern. Every parent should consider taking early control of and setting the ground rules for healthy sleep routines at an early stage in their child's life. This can begin around the time your child becomes aware of the difference between day and night. This usually happens between the ages of three and six months. Once this good, consistent sleep routine is in place, it is more than likely to create a good foundation for a life-long, successful sleeping pattern. The positive impact this will have on the child as well as their family far outweighs any feelings of guilt parents may experience about setting these rules for their children. The average child's day is filled with numerous opportunities for exploring and learning. These activities require energy in order to keep little bodies and brains functioning at their optimum level. Tired children are often cranky and irritable. The more tired these children become, the more emotionally dysfunctional their behavior is likely to be. Parents are reminded that no matter how exhausted your child may become while on the sleep-routine treadmill neither medication nor punishment is recommended for those who do not immediately fall asleep. Children may fight sleep because they are plagued by anxiety or fear or perhaps because they have been so hyped up during the day that they have trouble unwinding.

Children who enjoy sufficient restorative sleep have a more positive outlook on life. Their cognitive skills improve, and they cope better with problem-solving tasks and activities requiring creative thinking skills. These well-rested children demonstrate improved memory and the ability to learn new skills and recall information. With their increased energy levels, children who enjoy a good night's rest are more likely to make sensible, positive decisions. They are also better able to interact with others and generally enjoy good social relationships.

Sleep Deprivation

Parents should be alert to the signs of sleep deprivation in their children, which builds up surreptitiously over time. Continued disrupted sleep has been proven to adversely affect the area in the brain that handles reasoning and emotional responses. The result of too little sleep or poor-quality rest can have a far-reaching disastrous impact on the child's emotional, social, physical, and intellectual growth and development.

Sleep deprivation is a general term used to describe a consistent lack of sleep in an individual. The knock-on effect sleep deprivation in children has on their parents and siblings is likely to become an integral part of the increased stress levels of the entire family. According to Terry Cralle (n.d.), MS, RN, a recognized sleep educator, sleep deprivation can be a very stressful experience for both parents and children and is working to raise awareness of the problems this causes.

Sleep deprivation occurs when the child experiences consistent sleep disruption which occurs over a period of time. Staying awake longer than necessary causes the release of a chemical called cortisol. This chemical is detrimental to the body as it adversely affects the child's growth and their body's ability to heal and restore damaged cells and tissues.

When the body and mind are in a state of sleep deprivation, this is referred to as being in "sleep debt." The larger the debt, the more serious the negative impact on your child's capabilities, and the greater the increase in their behavioral, mental, and physical disorders. Eventually, symptoms may worsen and can result in severe depression or bipolar disorder. Genuine sleep disorders can be the result of illness or the use of medication. These disruptions may be short-lived if handled correctly and have no lasting effect on the child's long-term sleep routine. When left unchecked, sleep disorders may increase in momentum, becoming unmanageable.

Sleep Debt

Some people believe it is better to stay up late to complete a task, watch a movie, socialize, or read a book instead of going to bed at a reasonable time. Many adults find their workload demands late-night activity. Personal choice and poor sleep hygiene play an important role in sleep deprivation and the accumulation of sleep debt.

Sleep debt is the term used to describe the amount of sleep an individual lacks or has missed. People miss out on sleep for a variety of reasons. Sometimes illness and pain keep them awake. Other times their sleep patterns are disturbed by noise, temperature or insomnia (the inability to fall asleep). There are, however, those people who choose to stay awake for work, study of pleasure. Whatever the reason, a consistent lack of regular sleep is detrimental to our health. The greater our sleep debt, the less likely we are to recognize it. Perhaps this is due to the lifestyles to which we have become accustomed. A poem by Edna St Vincent Millay, entitled "My Candle Burns at Both Ends", sums up our modern lifestyle:

'My candle burns at both ends; it will not last the night,

But ah, my foes, and oh, my friends -

It gives a lovely light!'

Quiet Space

If it is at all possible, try to create the child's bedroom as their sanctuary, a safe and peaceful area in the home to which they can retreat for periods of solace and reflection. The bedroom should not be a social gathering place for friends and family unless of course the child is confined to bed for some medical reason. When a child identifies their bedroom or even their bed as their safe, quiet space, they will be more amenable to cooperating when sleep routines are put in place.

The Importance of "Pockets of Peace"

Living life in the fast lane brings with it an increased number of long hours, short periods of sleep, and the ever-present stress that accompanies this lifestyle.

A fundamental reason for sleep deprivation and all its associated negative psychological, social, health, and physical complications is stress. Although peace may appear to be an elusive quality of life, it behooves parents to assist their children in their search for "pockets of peace" in their everyday lives.

Peaceful spaces and actions enable the body to rest and restore its own energy. Many children enjoy the simple actions of lying on the freshly cut lawn or making snow angels on a wintery day.

Some children find peace in looking at the stars while others may enjoy tossing pebbles into a pond.

Older children may find solace in music, singing or dancing, or horseback riding with the wind blowing through their hair. Whatever their pocket of peace means to them, it is vitally important for the child's well-being that their parents provide opportunities for these peaceful interludes.

Resources for Parents

Parents are often in need of extra support and advice in one form or another. Time constraints during the day may prohibit the chance to meet with professional advisors face-to-face. Technology has developed an amazing variety of useful apps that may assist parents in their specific quest for support in establishing good sleep routines for their children, as well as being beneficial to themselves.

Some apps are purely music or sound oriented. These offer a wide variety of peaceful, soothing music and sound compilations that have a soporific effect on the brain, causing it to relax and encourage deep, restful sleep. Most of these apps have a timer that can be preset to turn off the sound after a specific time. There is also an option to allow the entire program to run, end-over-end, throughout the night. Some of these apps have a "wake-me-up" feature which can be adjusted by the user.

Other apps are in the form of calming, heart-warming bedtime stories for adults. These stories may be read by a male or female voice, depending on the choice of the listener. Each story is self-contained and is usually set in peaceful, calm surroundings. A great deal of calming adjectives and descriptive details are used throughout each story to create a visual picture for the listener. For adults who enjoy storytelling, these apps may prove beneficial in encouraging regular, restful, deep sleep.

The choices for app support are almost endless and will be dependent on the individual needs of the user. It may be a good idea to research what options are available and where possible, make use of FREE app options before you make a final choice.

Apps for Adults

Music and Meditation

Calming and soothing music and background sounds can be beneficial for both the parents and the child and may be used to set a positive, peaceful tone in the quiet space in preparation for bedtime.

Music, being an international language in its own right, carries its individual power to influence people across the globe. Some people have very definite music choices while others enjoy a more eclectic approach. Whatever your taste and preference, there is sure to be something among these options on offer that will appeal to your specific family and more importantly perhaps, to the child you are training into a good sleep routine. So, let's jump right into this space and view some of the many options available, in order to discover the perfect starting point for the creation of pockets of peace in your home.

Headspace: Meditation and Sleep

Headspace has created an innovative app that offers the user a well-structured beginner's course on how to develop personal mindfulness through meditation. Through the use of carefully selected soundtracks, created to encompass the listener in an all-enveloping sensation of peace and harmony, this app helps the user learn life-changing mindfulness, meditation, and relaxation skills that will have a long-lasting positive effect on aspects of life.

Mindfulness refers to the ability to exist purposefully and completely in the present. As the word implies, mindfulness encompasses alertness and conscious awareness of the entire environment, including all the sensory stimuli of sounds, sensations, smell, sight, and taste as well as the sixth area of sensory enlightenment, that of inner-personal perception.

Through consistent training and daily practice, mindfulness can have an overall positive outcome for many aspects of life. It can increase the production of endorphins, which will have numerous benefits from decreasing stress levels to improving the ability to focus and complete tasks.

This app, which is available from Amazon, may prove useful in assisting the parents and their children in discovering the magic of peaceful, guided meditation techniques that may have a lasting positive effect for good, restful sleep-training.

Comments

Parents and older children had a lot of positive comments to make about the Headspace app. They felt the meditation exercises gave them ample opportunity to relax and learn to control their own emotions. The results of their participation in the mindfulness sessions left them rested and more focused.

Noisli: Improve Focus and Boost Productivity

Noisli is an interesting app, available on Google Play and YouTube, that has created a multitude of environmental background sounds that may be applied singly or in any combination the user may choose.

It is believed these soundboards can assist concentration and improve focus as well as support relaxation by effectively drowning out the irritating, distracting cacophonous sounds of modern living.

Where previous generations lived in quiet solitude or enjoyed the soothing sounds of the daily hustle-and-bustle common at the time, modern humanity has become used to the increased noise level in most environments in the 21st century. Compared to modern children, those who lived in the 20th century and beyond were more in tune with their natural surroundings and fewer demands were made on their time. The Noisli app, which applies to everyday living, is multifunctional for smartphones as well as computers. The Noisli app offers online training.

Slumber: Fall Asleep and Insomnia App

The Slumber sleep app offers a very interesting alternate solution to sleep challenges. It consists of a wonderful variety of suitable, calming sleep-story paradigms that induce a sense of peace and harmony and encourage easy sleep. These dreamy stories encourage the brain to drift into a special, safe space in which we can reclaim some of our childhood joy and wonder. The Slumber app is offered on YouTube as well as Google Play.

Sleep Cycle: A Time App

Sleep Cycle is an iPhone app that works like a clock or timer. It functions by using the accelerometer, which detects and recognizes your movements during sleep. It is preprogrammed to use this data to wake you after a specific interval.

The app is dual purpose in that it not only acts as an alarm clock, but it also monitors sleep and provides daily feedback on this data.

This app is more suitable for adolescents and adults.

10% Happier: Meditation & Sleep

The 10% Happier app offers just that—the promise of making you feel at least 10% happier. How does this app work? Well, through guided talks and meditations, suitable videos, and sleep content, it aims to build and improve your meditation skills and boost these in order that you may enjoy better sleep routines as well as improved relationships.

The wide variety of options to choose from that give everyone who is interested in uplifting their mood and developing valuable mindfulness strategies encourage the daily use of this easily accessible app.

Pzizz: Sleep - Nap - Focus

The Pzizz app is the best App to hack your sleep and there is a FREE version available.

This app offers three important features: Sleep Feature Mode, Nap Feature Mode, and Focus Feature Mode.

The Pzizz app is easy and comfortable to use. Settings for each feature can be chosen, and time lapses are set to the individual's needs. The process involves a series of short meditation clips for napping and longer and more complex guided meditation for sleeping purposes. At the end of each segment and based on the programmed time-lapse, a voice prompt sounds as your wake-up alert.

A brand-new feature on Pzizz, the Focus Mode is very valuable when you require extra focus or concentration. This feature assists the brain in reaching an optimum functioning state, giving the user a much-needed boost of intellectual energy, as it were.

Apps for Children

Music, Songs, Educational Activities and Meditation

A wide variety of wonderful apps suitable for use with children is available to parents. Always remember to ensure the app is age-appropriate for your child and do some in-depth research before purchasing the final product.

Apps designed specifically for children focus on the material to which they will relate. Fantasy, exploration of new exciting topics, as well as fun and laughter often form the foundation for these music, story, or sound apps.

Breathe, Think, Do - 123 Sesame Street

This app is specifically designed to cater to children between the ages of two and five years of age. It is a story and sound app supported by jolly characters and lots of cheerful, catchy tunes and songs.

Breathe, Think, Do aims at assisting parents and caregivers with the support they need in teaching their children valuable problem-solving and planning skills as well as the ability to remain focused on a task until it reaches completion. There are also activities to promote auditory memory skills, language development, managing conflict situations, and developing self-control.

Comments

Children enjoy the interactive design of this app. They learned many of the songs and rhymes which helped them to relax.

Calm: Meditation & Sleep

Calm is an iPhone app specifically designed with guided meditation material to cater to those who require added support in order to fall into a deep, restful sleep. It offers the user the opportunity to divest the brain of all stress and tension, allowing it to declutter from the day's exhausting events and evolve into the magical creative organ it was designed to be.

Calm has developed a School Initiative which aims at introducing mindfulness into the school curriculum. Modern children desperately require added support, both at home and at school, if they are to live fully productive, happy lives because they live with unbelievable stress and demands, only some of a physical nature while others are of a social and emotional character. The negative, harmful impact of stress on the modern child has reached overwhelming proportions. This is very evident in the way these children behave and the serious level to which their accumulated academic successes have deteriorated.

Mindfulness, which has its roots in Eastern meditative practices, embraces the purposeful attention to the present moment with kindness, peacefulness and curiosity. Its objective is to instill this awareness into children in order for them to become aware of the importance and value of finding pockets of peace in their lives, spaces to which they can retreat in safety to replenish their mind, body, and soul. These moments of mindfulness offer the child the opportunity to "cultivate a stronger relationship" with themselves through becoming "in-tune" with their own body and inner self.

The practice of developing mindfulness in children differs vastly from that of adults. Children have an innate innocence that enables them to view the world with wonder and awe. Young children possess a matchless appreciation and passion for their world. These children can benefit from mindfulness training which can empower them to cope with the challenges of their everyday lives. The Calm app is available at iStores and YouTube

Comments

The Calm app proved to be a very popular app with older children who found it helpful for social conflict issues and improving self-confidence. It has offered the necessary support to children who require "pockets of peace" and the opportunity to escape from their hectic day. Calm has also helped children to focus better in the classroom.

Breathing Bubbles: Anxiety Release

The Breathing Bubbles app can be found on YouTube or on the Momentous Institute website.

The app is child-friendly and easy to operate. Once downloaded, your child can access the Breathing Bubbles app when they feel anxious or afraid.

The app displays a colorful screen in which a simple menu appears. The menu displays a variety of words, each referring to a negative feeling or concern the child may have. So for example, if the child feels afraid, they press the relevant bubble icon, which then floats away. The instruction to the child is to breathe deeply as the icon fades.

The positive implications for the child using the Breathing Bubbles app are that the easy to use format empowers the child to find potential support when they need it. Although the app is easy for a child to use, positive adult reinforcement will be required to add support and give the child the opportunity to talk about his feelings.

Comments

The Breathing Bubbles app is popular with the younger children in elementary school in helping them overcome emotional challenges of sadness, anger and frustration. The Breathing Bubbles has a calming effect on these children which helps them to focus on positive issues and to re-organize their thoughts. It's a sort of "time-out" opportunity.

Stop, Breathe and Think Kid: Meditation and Self-Help

The Stop, Breathe and Think Kid app on YouTube offers a wide variety of apps to support children in need of some much-needed quiet time.

This kids mindfulness app takes the form of lovely, imaginative stories suitable for children between the ages of four to six years.

Each story involves a gentle, loving, and protective companion in the form of "Bulldog" that travels through with the child. There are lots of repetitive breathing activities included in each story. The child is encouraged to follow the simple instructions to relax and focus on specific information given by the soporific voice on the app. In next to no time, the child begins to drop off to sleep in a safe, quiet, happy environment.

Parents may also find added ideas and information from Kids Mindfulness: Calm or Kids Mindfulness: Games for Sleep to assist them in developing a consistent, peaceful sleep routine for their children.

What kids have to say about this app

Children between the ages of five and six years who used this kids mindfulness app reported they enjoyed the stories and felt well-rested when they awoke the following morning.

The Stop, Breathe and Think Kid app relaxes the user and affords them the chance to drift off easily into a restful sleep.

Kids Yoga Deck: Body Relaxation and Peace of Mind - Molly Schreiber

Molly Schreiber (Schreiber, n.d.), makes use of a series of well-presented Yoga cards each displaying a specific Yoga pose for the child to see and mimic. Each card has the name of the pose printed in both English and Sanskrit.

Yoga offers the child an opportunity to stretch and strengthen their body muscles in a gentle, controlled manner while learning to use breathing techniques to improve the absorption of oxygen in the body.

Yoga exercises that are done before bedtime can be most beneficial to children with sleep disorders. Through these exercises, the children develop the ability to relax both their mind and body.

Smiling Minds: Meditation for Kids

The Smiling Minds app has been adapted for older children of school-going age. It offers emotional support to children who are struggling to cope with sadness, loneliness, emotional fatigue, and social challenges.

In some schools in the United States, Smiling Minds: Meditation for Kids, has been introduced as part of the curriculum. This app has proven beneficial to many children as it gives them a well-defined quiet space in which they can calm down and rethink their best course of action. By making use of this app there may be fewer emotional outbursts, which will in turn assist in the development of improved social relationships. Smiling Minds: Meditation for Kids may also be beneficial to the development of good, individual coping mechanisms.

Mindfulness training helps children to focus on the present. The human brain is full of information, particularly past information. Mindfulness training develops mental skills that help the child take control of their brain instead of the other way around.

When the brain takes control of our thoughts, it either forces us into past situations by recalling memories of incidents that have already occurred, or it pushes our thoughts toward the future possibilities that may happen. With this "running around" process in our brain, we can become very anxious. We recall past information like a fight or a falling-out with a friend. The negative residue of the feelings we experienced at that time resurface and renew the anxiety or sadness we experienced. This brain activity causes undue stress and anxiety for the child.

Children who benefit from mindfulness training develop an increased awareness of their own strengths and how to put these to good use with beneficial results for themselves as well as others. Mindfulness training helps children to identify their weaknesses and use positive behavior strategies to overcome these. The Smiling Mind: Meditation for Kids app is available on YouTube.

Sleep Gadgets to Help Your Child Fall Asleep

A wonderful variety of modern technological gadgets are now available to assist and support parents in their efforts to develop good sleep routines for their children. A good night's sleep in some households is a rare event. So, to assist you in your search for the elusive solution to the very real problem of sleepless children, here are some ideas.

Hatch Baby Rest

Hatch Baby Rest is a delightful, color-changing bedside lamp specifically designed for children.

The Hatch Baby Rest lamp comes fitted with a high-quality speaker that can be remotely controlled by the parents via the cell phone app. It emits soothing white noise and changes color throughout the night.

Reports indicate the Hatch Baby Rest lamp, which is obtainable from Amazon, is a popular accessory for bedrooms for children between the age of six months to around eight years.

What parents have to say about this gadget

Hatch Baby Rest is an attractive, functional, value-for-money night light. The white noise is pleasantly soothing.

Zazu Kids

Zazu Kids are the manufacturers of, among many other night lights and sleep gadgets for children, the following three delightfully innovative gadgets.

- Pam the Penguin is a bedside light fitted with a wireless Bluetooth speaker. The little lamp burns through the night changing to orange 30 minutes before the child's scheduled wake-up time. It then turns green to indicate the day has begun and the child is ready to go.

- Bobby the Bear is an all-in-one analog-digital clock suitable for older children who are learning to tell the time. The bear closes its eyes at night to indicate the time for bed and reopens them in the morning.

- Lou the Owl is a night light with an adjustable-brightness option ideal for those little ones who are fearful of the dark.

What parents have to say about these gadgets

These gadgets are attractive and functional. They are available from takealot.com. Bobby the Bear all-in-one digital clock will be a useful tool for teaching young children the time.

Smart Connect Deluxe Soother

This is an all-in-one Fisher-Price gadget with a multifunctional sound-light that shines through a beautifully designed shade, projecting stars on silhouettes on the wall and emitting a soft, comforting glow from the base of the lamp. The lamp plays soothing music and white noise which can be controlled via an app. Available from Amazon.

What parents have to say about this gadget

The Smart Connect Deluxe Soother may be your best buy ever as the device to get your child's bedtime routine off to a positive start.

Cozy Phones

These upbeat electronic gadgets come with a colorful headband fitted with tiny earphones for easy comfort. Children can listen to their favorite sleep music as they drift off to dreamland.

What parents have to say about this gadget

This delightful, inventive and easy-to-use sleep training gadget may well prove its usefulness for older children to help them to develop healthy sleep habits.

The Dodow

The Dodow is an interesting example of technology that has been developed to shine an expanding and contracting blue light on the ceiling to which the child breathes rhythmically in and out. This may be a good option for older children who have difficulty unwinding after their busy day.

Serenity Star

The Serenity Star is a combination light-sound clock device with a built-in temperature sensor that changes color when the room is too hot or cold and is made by the designers and developers, aden-anais. Running off either plug-in or battery power it plays a variety of lullabies, white noise, and even the sound of a heartbeat.

What parents have to say about this gadget

Parents will find The Serenity Star plays a lovely, peaceful selection of well-known lullabies that are suitable for young children. The light emitted is sufficient for nighttime routines feeds and diaper changes.

The Final Choice

The apps and gadgets mentioned in this book are only a minute selection of the myriad of options available.

As far as possible the information researched on this selection of items has been gathered from reliable sources and has been presented in a fair and unbiased manner. No personal preferences of the author or editor have been included.

As with all things, the final choice is a personal one, based on the individual preferences of the parents and the sleep temperament of their children.

References

American Academy of Pediatrics. (2014). Let them sleep: AAP recommends delaying start times of middle and high schools to combat teen sleep deprivation. Retrieved from https://www.aap.org/en-us/about-the-aap/aap-press-room/Pages/Let-Them-Sleep-AAP-Recommends-Delaying-Start-Times-of-Middle-and-High-Schools-to-Combat-Teen-Sleep-Deprivation.aspx

American Academy of Pediatrics. (2016). American Academy of Pediatrics supports childhood sleep guidelines. (2016). Retrieved from https://www.aap.org/en-us/about-the-aap/aap-press-room/Pages/American-Academy-of-Pediatrics-Supports-Childhood-Sleep-Guidelines.aspx

American Academy of Pediatrics. (n.d.) Ages & stages. Retrieved from https://www.healthychildren.org/English/ages-stages/Pages/default.aspx

American Academy of Pediatrics. (n.d.) Brush, book, bed: How to structure your child's nighttime routine. Retrieved from https://www.healthychildren.org/English/healthy-living/oral-health/Pages/Brush-Book-Bed.aspx/

BabySparks. (2017). Instilling good sleep habits in your baby. Retrieved from https://babysparks.com/2017/03/03/instilling-good-sleep-habits-for-your-baby/

BrightHorizons. (n.d.). What is my parenting style? Four types of parenting. Retrieved from https://www.brighthorizons.com/family-resources/parenting-style-four-types-of-parenting

Brown, M. (2016). Here are just a few of the crazy things that happen when you're a sleep-deprived parent. Retrieved from https://www.cosmopolitan.com/health-fitness/news/a57135/sleep-deprived-parenting-stories/

Cralle, T. (n.d.). Books. Retrieved from http://www.terrycralle.com/books/

DeJeu, E. (2019). Healthy sleep habits, happy child: Our review. Retrieved from https://www.babysleepsite.com/sleep-training/healthy-sleep-habits-happy-child-review/

Ferber, R. (2006). *Resolve your child's sleep problems.* New York, NY: Touchstone.

Fuller, C., Lehman, E., Hicks, S., & Novick, M. (2017). bedtime use of technology and associated sleep problems in children. *Global Pediatric Health, 4.* doi: 10.1177/2333794X17736972

Gamsky, J. (2016). Why is sleep so important for students? Retrieved from https://www.uatutoring.com/blog/2016/7/1/why-is-sleep-so-important-for-students

Gerber, L. (2014). Sleep deprivation in children: A growing public health concern. *Nursing Management, (45)*, 8, 22-28.

Henderson, R. (2016). Psychosomatic disorders. Retrieved from https://patient.info/mental-health/psychosomatic-disorders

Hochron, A. (2016). Kimberly Hardin: Differentiating between sleep disorders and finding best treatments. Retrieved from https://www.mdmag.com/medical-news/kimberly-hardin-differentiating-between-sleep-disorders-and-finding-best-treatments

Holt, L. E. (1907). *The care and feeding of children.* New York, NY: D. Appleton & Co. As retrieved from https://www.gutenberg.org/files/15484/15484-h/15484-h.htm

https://www.gerberfoundation.org/focus-areas/

https://www.sleepfoundation.org/sleep-topics/children-teens-sleep

https://www.smilingmind.com.au/

Hurley, K. (n.d.). Is it sleep deprivation or depression? Retrieved from https://www.psycom.net/sleep-deprivation-depression

IQ Test Experts. (n.d.) Rubik's cube improves spatial IQ. Retrieved from https://www.iqtestexperts.com/iq-sleep.php

Johnson, N. (2019a). Baby sleep needs by age. Retrieved from https://www.babysleepsite.com/baby-sleep-needs/baby-sleep-needs-by-age/

Johnson, N. (2019b). Ferber or Weissbluth? Retrieved from https://www.babysleepsite.com/sleep-training/ferber-or-weissbluth/

Kovac, S. (2018). Gadgets that help kids fall asleep and stay asleep. Retrieved from https://www.pcmag.com/feature/362600/gadgets-that-help-kids-fall-asleep-and-stay-asleep

McGurgan, H., & Kania, J. (2018). Understanding delayed growth and how it's treated. Retrieved from https://www.healthline.com/health/delayed-growth-symptom

Michigan Medicine. (n.d.). Sleep problems. Retrieved from http://www.med.umich.edu/yourchild/topics/sleep.htm

National Sleep Foundation. (n.d.). Healthy sleep tips. Retrieved from https://www.sleepfoundation.org/articles/healthy-sleep-tips

Parenting for Brain. (2019). 4 parenting styles – Characteristics and effects. Retrieved from https://www.parentingforbrain.com/4-baumrind-parenting-styles/

Positive-Parenting-Ally. (n.d.). Diana Baumrind's 3 parenting styles: Get a full understanding of the 3 archetypical parents. Retrieved from https://www.positive-parenting-ally.com/3-parenting-styles.html

Rapaport, L., (2017). Lack of sleep tied to higher risk of diabetes in kids. Retrieved from https://www.reuters.com/article/us-health-children-sleep-diabetes/lack-of-sleep-tied-to-higher-risk-of-diabetes-in-kids-idUSKCN1AV1S5

Research Gate. (n.d.). Sumi Rose. Retrieved from https://www.researchgate.net/profile/Sumi_Rose

Rockefeller University Press. (2019). How sleep can fight infection. Retrieved from https://www.sciencedaily.com/releases/2019/02/190212094839.htm

Rosenthal, M. (2009). The 4 parenting styles: What works and what doesn't. Retrieved from http://theattachedfamily.com/?p=2151

Schreiber, M. (n.d.). About Molly Schreiber. Retrieved from https://www.yogaalliance.org/TeacherPublicProfile?tid=98596

Scientific American. (2015). What happens in the brain during sleep? Retrieved from https://www.scientificamerican.com/article/what-happens-in-the-brain-during-sleep1/

Sleep debt. (n.d.) In *Wikipedia*. Retrieved from https://en.wikipedia.org/wiki/Sleep_debt[KL7]

Stanford Health Care. (n.d.). Pediatric sleep disorders. Retrieved from https://stanfordhealthcare.org/medical-conditions/sleep/pediatric-sleep-disorders.html - Nov 2019

Tedesco, S., & Lake Abdelrahman, A. (2019). 7 best sleep apps to download in 2019, according to experts. Retrieved from https://www.goodhousekeeping.com/health/wellness/g26963663/best-sleep-apps/

The Douglas Research Centre. (n.d.). Sleep and children: The impact of lack of sleep on daily life. Retrieved from https://douglas.research.mcgill.ca/sleep-and-children-impact-lack-sleep-daily-life

The University of Kansas Health System. (n.d.). Sleep Disorders. Retrieved from https://www.kansashealthsystem.com/care/specialties/sleep-disorders

Thompson, K., & Fogel, S. (2019). Simultaneous EEG-fMRI reveals neural substrates during sleep that support Fluid Intelligence. Retrieved from https://pressrelease.brainproducts.com/eeg-fmri-during-sleep/

Timmons, J. (2016). Does the pick up, put down method work to get your baby to sleep? Retrieved from https://www.healthline.com/health/parenting/pick-up-put-down-method

Tuck Sleep. (2019). Stages of sleep and sleep cycles. Retrieved from https://www.tuck.com/stages/

WebMD. (n.d.). Sleep problems in children. Retrieved from https://www.webmd.com/sleep-disorders/guide/children-sleep-problems

Weissbluth, M. (2015). *Healthy sleep habits, happy child, 4th edition: A step-by-step program for a good night's sleep.* New York, NY: Ballantine Books.

Wu, L., and Van Kaer, L. (2011). Natural killer T cells in health and disease. *Frontiers in Bioscience, 3,* 236-251.

Zeidman, A. (2018). The 8 best sleep apps and meditation apps that relax kids. Retrieved from https://www.fatherly.com/gear/best-sleep-apps-kids/

www.ingramcontent.com/pod-product-compliance
Lightning Source LLC
Chambersburg PA
CBHW071519080526
44588CB00011B/1489